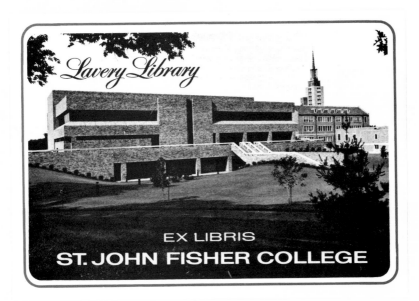

Working with the Elderly

Golden Age Books
Perspective on Aging

Series Editor: Steven L. Mitchell

Working with the Elderly

An Introduction

edited by

Elizabeth S. Deichman, Ed.M., OTR

and

Regina Kociecki, B.A.

Prometheus Books
Buffalo, New York

Published 1989 by Prometheus Books
700 East Amherst Street, Buffalo, New York 14215
Copyright © 1989 by Elizabeth S. Deichman and Regina Kociecki

Library of Congress Cataloging-in-Publication Data
Working with the elderly.

(Golden age books)
Includes bibliographical references.
1. Social work with the aged. I. Deichman,
Elizabeth S. II. Kociecki, Regina. III. Series.
HV1451.W66   1989   362.6   89-10856
ISBN 0-87975-520-2
ISBN 0-87975-534-2 (pbk.)

Printed in the United States of America

Foreword

Welcome to your future—perhaps the last social frontier: the fascinating world of gerontology. It is a relatively new discipline, with formal organization of its many service providers and scholars having taken place under the aegis of the Gerontological Association only in the late 1940s.

After the Second World War, the knowledge explosion—followed by improved living standards, sanitation, and medical care—found Americans confounding the actuarial tables—they were living much longer than they were expected to. Up to that point gerontologists used a Band-Aid approach to problems. This is no longer acceptable—it is inefficient, insufficient, and wasteful. Now a mass of knowledge has been accumulated, statistical data have been collected and analyzed by computers in dozens of combinations and hundreds of variations, inferences have been drawn, and activist groups have emerged and joined the fray. Social engineering has begun in earnest. We truly have come a long way since the Social Security Act of 1935.

The coming generation of seniors may well be their own social architects in an increasingly pluralistic society. With this text we hope to introduce some of the many dimensions of the multitude of concerns of the present. The present and past experiences are the foundation for developing new strategies, new lifestyles, new knowledge and ideas. Let Star Wars begin with your vision for a utopian old age. Why not? It's *your* old age we're talking about!

Contents

8   Contents

1

The Challenge of Aging

Elizabeth S. Deichman and Regina Kociecki

There are those whom time can never age—not even with years.
These keep a dream, not let its flame burn low . . .

They look ahead, beyond regrets and tears—
Old Age is something they can never know.

—Margaret E. Bruner

In your mind, slowly walk down the corridor of a nursing home: you become conscious of eyes following you, yet soon you are aware that some eyes don't "see" you. Hands may reach out to you for human contact—any human touch, even a stranger's. It seems the corridor is filled with wheelchairs: frail bodies slumped and restrained, surely uncomfortable if not in pain. Margaret Bruner's words have a hollow, empty ring, don't they? But do we really *know* that? Perhaps the eyes that seem so vacant are on a journey to a distant time, reliving a happier and more pleasant occasion, unaware of the restraints on the body, unaware of pain. "Yes, but . . . I wouldn't want to live so long, under those conditions." We've said it, others have echoed it, and at some point you may voice similar impressions. Since the fact is that less than 5 percent of the elderly will find themselves in such a state of precarious health and dependence, why this negative, almost fatalistic expectation? "Human nature," we suppose.

If so, we can take lessons from an "average" American, Mary Vieillard—pianist, housewife, and mother. In a delightful book, which she wrote at

9

the age of ninety-four, she describes how a serious back injury at age eighty-four forced her to give up her comfortable apartment and make a "home" in four different nursing homes during the next ten years. The book is aptly titled *It Is Not as Late as You Think*. In an introductory paragraph she writes, "We must keep doors open to opportunities for mental expansion, continuing to participate in the world of interests and not become shriveled souls with unmindful attitudes toward life."

In those four nursing homes, did Mary Vieillard find easy and obvious solutions? Not at all. She writes that first she was forced to draw on her own spiritual and mental resources to discover compassion for those physically and mentally less active and alert than herself. She learned to mingle with her new neighbors and even to communicate in new ways—with a nod of the head, a pat, and an attentive attitude. She willed herself to develop composure and poise to overcome petty annoyances and irritations in dealing with administrators, nurses, and other residents.

In her eighty-fifth year Ms. Vieillard became a correspondent for a local newspaper, and learned the mechanics of playing a Wurlitzer organ! Her music instructor was twenty-two. At ninety-one she tackled public speaking when she was invited to address a conference of professionals in the field of aging. Of her ten years in four nursing homes Ms. Vieillard observed, "Through keeping a flexible mind and an open heart, I am learning the lessons of patience, tolerance, and compassion and am gradually reaching self-actualization and fulfillment as a human being." Please note that, at age ninety-four, Ms. Vieillard wrote in the present, active tense.

Throughout this short treatise her vibrant philosophy on personal responsibility inspires. It even overcomes the negative and superficial reactions to that mental journey down the nursing home corridor. Ultimately, Ms. Vieillard suggests that we alone are responsible for the personal view of our life experiences.

It is incumbent then on the individual to prepare responsibly and as realistically as possible for those last decades of life. True, some of life's traumas are beyond personal control. Much of life is little more than being at the right place at the right time—luck, if you will. But we can discipline ourselves throughout life to develop the flexibility and optimistic outlook that are of great importance in successful aging.

The ability to be open to new situations and to cope with challenges is an extension of the educational process. When we speak of education, most of us visualize a classroom filled with eager shining young faces. Education, however, comes in many forms, and the traditional classroom is but the beginning of a process that continues throughout life, whether we are conscious of it or not. The traditional classroom introduces us merely to the basics, but the complexities of modern life demand much more of us than mere basics, whether it be in mathematics, English, sociology, technology, or whatever. These days academicians are debating whether the baccalaureate degree is obsolete, like the dodo bird. The need for constant retraining and upgrading is foreseen as new occupations emerge and/or become more sophisticated. In certain professions—medicine and engineering, for example—continuing education has been a fact for decades and is a requirement for continued licensing and/or certification.

The great experiment in lifelong education is beginning to include elderly citizens. They are encouraged to learn new skills and develop new hobbies, to rekindle old interests and sharpen minds in a variety of ways and places. American highways are filled with busloads of seniors, crisscrossing the country, discovering this vast land and its treasures, not as armchair travelers but breathing, eating, feeling, and seeing firsthand its diversity. These excursions are a shot in the arm for the travel industry. Senior centers are filled with activities: from ethnic cooking classes to the beat of the cha-cha-cha as participants limber up with aerobic exercises. Seniors are invited to audit courses free of charge at public colleges. They register for moderately priced mini courses in a nationwide Elderhostel program whose popularity has mushroomed beyond the founder's expectation.

Social scientists are developing studies to learn what keeps eighty-year-olds going and to see what we can learn from them to help others. "One reason to study these people is because they're successes," says psychologist Marion Perlmutter. "If you can make it to eighty, you're doing something right." Preliminary interviews suggest that "the ability to be open to new situations and to cope with challenges distinguish people who grow during adulthood from people who stabilize or decline," she comments.

There are many different ways of learning and a universe full of things to learn about. We have the capacity to learn from reading books, watching television, discussions with friends, as well as sitting in a classroom. We're familiar with the "school of hard knocks," which is just another way of saying, "experience is the best teacher—she tests first and teaches afterward." If, like author Vieillard, we can observe, analyze, react, and translate our life experiences into a less stressful and more compassionate existence, and if we add to the quality of our lives with new knowledge—and new friends—then we can assert that we are truly lifelong learners.

What are the advantages of informal versus formal learning situations? Why go back to the classroom—a situation many of us don't always recall with pleasure. Learning informally and individually, we can hop, skip, and jump from subject to subject at whatever pace we choose, wherever and whenever we elect to do so. Classroom learning, on the other hand, finds us committed to exploring a topic at some depth for a fixed period of time—six, ten, fifteen weeks—with a group as diverse in background as is seldom found even in our pluralistic society. There is an instructor, skilled in guiding inquiries, who keeps the group from digressing too far afield. If the class is representative and fortunate enough to match our pluralistic society, there will be people of assorted ages, races, ethnic mixtures, as well as those of different socioeconomic groups. Such broad exposure to diverse experiences and outlooks is not available in our social or work life where we usually seek out those with similar interests and points of view.

What age would you choose if you could set your chronological clock either backward or forward? Perhaps you feel, as we do, that "the best age to be is the age you are now." This popular bumper sticker slogan expresses a realistic attitude that enables those who live by it not to fritter away the present, wishing to change the unchangeable.

In a recent address, Dr. Perry Gresham, author and well-known advocate of creative aging, said, "Life is a series of renewals rather than a machine that wears out a little at a time." Ponce de Leon should have searched for the "Fountain of Age," which he could have found within himself. These "new ideas" about old age are the subject of Dr. Gresham's book *With Wings as Eagles.* According to Gresham, there are three philosophies from which a person can choose an attitude toward aging. The first one is called "the old car" theory in which the body and mind gradually break down in all the parts until they are finally useless. This attitude holds out no hope or encouragement of anything better. A second attitude, called "the old tree" image, is probably the most widely held today. In this theory, human life is regarded as vegetation that springs up (youth), matures (summer), grows old (autumn), and dies (winter) as the seasons turn.

Gresham, a former university dean, says that he held this view of aging along with most people until he personally became aware of a surge of renewed energy when he entered his sixties. He agreed with Henri Bergson, a French philosopher who said, "For a conscious being to exist is to change, to change is to mature, to mature is to go on creating one's self endlessly."

This is the basis for the third theory: the surge of energy necessary for a mature eagle's initial flight is there when it is required. Gresham says that if there is work that a person wants to do, the energy required will surge up no matter what the age. Man has a resurgence of strength three or four times in his life—each time to meet the demands of the moment. The demands made in the later years of life are as challenging and as likely to be met with the necessary surge of energy as at any other time of life.

There is a period of renewal in later life. Gresham supports this theory, not only from his own experience, but also from the evidence gained from the accomplishments of such famous elders as Plato, Benjamin Franklin,

Pablo Picasso, Albert Schweitzer, and Arthur Fiedler. All of them were prodigious creators, each produced even more prolifically in later years.

This period of renewal can be particularly meaningful in our increasingly multigenerational society. Dr. Arthur Korhaber, a psychiatrist and coauthor of *Grandparents/Grandchildren: The Vital Connection,* feels strongly that the very young and the very old go together naturally, so much so that youngsters without grandparents will oftentimes "adopt" some. He says old people serve special purposes for the young—e.g., living ancestor, historian, nurturer, and role model.

Interesting arrangements between retirement homes and child day care centers are evolving, providing for instant grandparents and grandchildren. John Thompson, administrator of such a home in Buffalo, Minnesota, says, "As hard as we try to keep our residents active and alert, these kids do a better job just doing what kids do. Their life, youth, and energy keeps everybody stimulated. What children are looking for is a hug, a lap, a kind word, a touch, somebody to read a story, to smile and to share with." By encouraging this bond, we will build and foster respect for age and a better future for all.

Introductory sociology courses have long taught that humans have basic needs: food, clothing, shelter, love, safety. Gerontologists from the University of Iowa Institute on Gerontology expanded and identified "needs for a fuller life":

The need to render some socially useful service.

The need to be considered part of the community.

The need to enjoy normal companionship.

The need for recognition as an individual.

The need for opportunity for self-expression and a sense of achievement.

The need for health protection and care.

The need for suitable mental stimulation.

The need for suitable living arrangements and family relationships.

The need for spiritual satisfaction.

Examining these needs, we will note that to a great degree most of them are developed within the social milieu. Man is indeed a social being; he needs the stimulation and reinforcement of his contemporaries because they have lived through similar periods and experiences. Thus, an innovative program, Peer Counseling for the Elderly at the University of California, uses trained paraprofessionals, ages fifty-five to eighty-one, in offering counseling to older people.

Throughout the country, we find the beginnings of new social ventures that must to some degree replace the vanishing nuclear family: in New York City, seniors and teenagers team up to deliver groceries, clean house, chat, and reach out to the homebound; the Gray Panthers' pioneering experiments with in-home intergenerational living arrangements. We need to encourage such cooperation and programs to gain mutual understanding rather than wait with trepidation for the gloomy predictions of generational conflicts to come to pass.

The resources for fuller lives are within us but to a great extent they must be developed in the broader society—schools, offices, factories, churches, clubs, organizations, and governments. The world grows smaller every day and flexibility will be needed to meet the challenges ahead. The challenges will come from living in close quarters on an already crowded planet with people from every nationality, race, and socioeconomic status. Challenges successfully met, things learned, skills developed, and hobbies enjoyed at every age are all part of our personal package of resources that becomes larger with each passing year. Because it is probable that we will live some years after formal retirement, it is important to think clearly about what we will retire *to* as well as *from*. The resource package assembled in the years from birth to retirement will determine the direction we take.

The contents of the resource package will vary from person to person. Some will have the greatest resource of all—good health, with a body that will service its owner well. Health in later life depends on how we have nourished and exercised our bodies throughout the years.

Attitudes are also part of the resource package. Pessimism or optimism will play a large part in whether we wither or continue to grow in later years. "Can do" attitudes and helpful ideas promote positive growth. Former President Jimmy Carter and wife, Rosalynn, are not "average Americans" by any means. In 1980, after a stunning defeat at the hands of Ronald Reagan, the Carters were deeply in debt and traumatized by the repudiation of the American people. In *Everything to Gain: Making the Most of the Rest of Your Life,* they describe their experiences as they sought to remake their lives. Particularly interesting was their involvement as carpenters and laborers in "Habitat," an intergenerational effort to rebuild substandard housing for sale to low-income families. Jimmy and Rosalynn Carter were able to continue "giving," albeit on a different level, to a society that seemingly rejected them. As an observer during recent Panamanian national elections, the former president's keen and unbiased comments drew worldwide praise and "elder statesman" recognition at home.

Support groups of family and friends, new and old, are important parts of the resource package, as are the lifelong habits of reaching out to others for help.

Hobbies and interests acquired through the years are also part of the resource package. Explore the wealth of possibilities available at every age to find what recreations you enjoy.

The final piece in the package is money. This takes planning. Achieving financial security will free both mind and spirit to enable you to enjoy these special, later years to their fullest. A package of resources, well stocked, will serve you well on the journey to "The Fountain of Age."

Students of today are the change agents of the future. Theirs is the challenge of ever-escalating expectations for an improved quality of life in a rapidly changing and increasingly complex world. Their degree of success will be a reflection not only of the fundamental knowledge base provided by our educational establishment but also of the creative forces nurtured and unleashed in the learning processes.

In Biblical times the average lifespan was less than thirty years. Today, some 2,000 years later, as individuals we try to untangle the interpersonal relations of four and five generations coping with family responsibilities. As a society, in the midst of the Information Age, we try to control our destinies with a secure and viable future by peering into the tangle of demographics and technological innovations, preparing for a vastly larger elderly population living well past ninety and even overtaking the century mark.

The lifestyle of the present senior generation was molded by the social and economic upheavals of the Great Depression and World War II. They are the first-generation recipients of social services developed as a result of lessened familial responsibilities and replaced by government legislation. The trial-and-error, hit-or-miss evolution of some of these institutions and services is a matter of record. The old nursing home, a potential fire trap housed in a Victorian mansion and run by well-meaning but untrained amateurs, is history in most of the nation. It has been replaced with a carefully designed skilled nursing facility orchestrated to government specifications requiring x-number of square feet for each client to accommodate each specific activity.

Will present institutions and services be acceptable, adequate, or relevant to the modern Yuppie, weaned on health and fitness, well educated and traveled, whose body has been repaired with spare parts, plastic joints, artificial implants?

People are living longer, and they expect the quality of their life experiences to improve. They demand that their health care, their social lives, their entertainment, and their education reflect the improvements and variety enjoyed by the general population. In a service-oriented society, premium quality of service is increasingly viewed as a right.

The electronic era has ushered in the Information Age. But information by itself is an unread, unopened book or undecoded jargon scattered on a floppy disk. Information shared with one another and effectively applied is the essence of efficient communication—the basis of quality service. In this volume we hope to succeed in acquainting readers with some of the present-day services and practices as well as the major medical, social, legal, and ethical questions they pose to each of us who have dedicated our lives to the elderly. With this information, we hope service providers will strive to gain an understanding of the multi-faceted concerns of the various professionals with whom they may be working to build a better society. That society is us: readers, writers, planners, service providers, and consumers. Through an exchange of knowledge we can all learn to communicate our desires, our needs, and our dreams for what should be a delightful period of life, those twilight years, that will provide both fulfillment and a pathway for others to follow.

Communication is an art form in itself, as many of the authors point out. It includes body language, speech, touch, the written word, and activities. Communication processes, thoughtfully applied, build an initial climate of trust that enables self-actualization and fulfillment of mutual client/professional goals. The art of mutually participatory conversation must be continually practiced, honed, and analyzed before it can become an automatic, effective essence of the human being struggling, searching, and reaching for responses to questions and problems that challenge the aging individual in an aging society. There are no spectators when it comes to aging . . .

> Age is opportunity no less
> Than youth itself, though in another dress.
> And as the evening twilight fades away,
> The sky is filled with stars invisible by day.
>
> —Henry Wadsworth Longfellow

FOR DISCUSSION

1. Bring in two obituaries, one that you found interesting and another less appealing. Remember that obituaries are usually prepared by the family or, in the case of a public figure, by the press. Discuss points that held your interest or "turned you off" and explain why.

2. List three personality traits that you consider essential in working with the elderly on a one-to-one basis. List three personal attributes you would consider helpful when working in the field of aging in a teaching, planning, or administrative capacity.
3. What appeal, if any, does the field of aging have for you? Please explain.
4. List three of the most important problems you feel society faces in the field of aging during the next twenty-five years. Do you plan to be part of the solution? If so, in what capacity? Please explain.

BIBLIOGRAPHY

Carter, J., and Carter, R. *Everything to Gain: Making the Most of the Rest of Your Life.* New York: Fawcett, 1987.

Gresham, P. *With Wings as Eagles.* Winter Park, Fla.: Anna Publishing Inc., 1980.

Korhaber, A., and Woodward, K. *Grandparents/Grandchildren: The Vital Connection.* New York: Doubleday, 1984.

Vieillard, M. *It's Not as Late as You Think.* Buffalo, N.Y.: Potentials Development, 1980.

2

The Art of Communication: The Basis for Service

Dellvina Gross

As we become a closer, more densely populated world of older people, the art of communication is urgently needed to facilitate positive interaction, understanding, and peace. Human communication is certainly complex, yet absolutely crucial for survival. An intricate network of individual, cultural, linguistic and related factors enter into what appears to be a simple interaction between two people. How often do we hear, "There's obviously a communication problem in this situation . . ." or "He just can't communicate." Perhaps, the more amazing thing is that we so often do manage to communicate.

DEFINITIONS AND MODELS OF COMMUNICATION

In this chapter we define communication as "shared meaning." In other words, what the speaker says—words, intentions, inflections, and nonverbal verifications—is expressed within the same social context as the person receiving the message. The meaning of the communication, thus, is experienced in the same manner by both the speaker and the receiver or listener. This sharing is based upon mutual understanding of symbols, meanings, shared beliefs, attitudes, values, and life experiences.

We will look at communication models, principles, and concepts as

19

they facilitate the development of helping relationships with the elderly. Cross-cultural communication concepts in particular will be explored since the older person in our society has communicated across culture, ethnicity, race, religion, and geographic region through decades of varying life experiences. In the area of transportation, for example, changes occurring in the life of a seventy- or eighty-year-old person include going from horse-drawn vehicles to space shuttles. We have become a much smaller world: the relative isolation of a century or more ago that found most people living in one community or on one street for a lifetime has evolved to the highly mobile society of today, in which we travel across the country or around the world at any time. In addition, changes in financial and political circles are communicated almost instantaneously across national boundaries.

The purposes of communication are threefold: to inform, to persuade, and to entertain. Thus, we communicate in order to obtain understanding, agreement, and attraction. There must necessarily be agreement on the meaning of the words and symbols used and on the context to which that meaning applies, in order for mutual communication to occur. A commonality in backgrounds presupposes similarity in beliefs, attitudes and values, and an assumption that both parties are coming from the same place. This shared basis of life experiences promotes and facilitates a willingness to interact, to believe and to continue to communicate with one another.

The most universally understood communication model, that of David Berlo, has four components: the speaker, the message, the channel, and the receiver. Berlo also discusses the importance of feedback, listening, and individual interpretation. Another communication model, that of Frank Dance, shows environmental impact in his helical model in which the process is constantly changing, spiraling, with each interaction and feedback ongoing/changing/modifying and building upon the last communication. Catherine Galvin has a circular interpersonal communication model: the inner circle includes speaker/receiver attitudes as affected by (1) the occasion, which includes reason, time, and place; (2) content, including topic and material; and (3) organization of ideas and words. In her outer circle she lists attitudes indicated verbally by voice and articulation, and nonverbally by gestures, eye contact, and facial expression. Physical and social components that affect our ability to receive and interpret communication are included: e.g., age, race, sex, dress, mannerism, titles, background, personality, occupation, education, economic status, and culture. Feedback and interference are indicated as ongoing processes that are constantly present and affect the interactions.

Returning to Berlo's four major components, let us reflect briefly upon the channels of communication used to convey a message. These may determine who the receivers are, who listens to which radio station or television program, who prefers reading, as well as who uses and is more influenced by oral communication. Many cultures, including those of Africa, communicate orally from generation to generation via stories. Thus history, beliefs, attitudes, and values are communicated by word of mouth using nonverbal elaboration—music, song, rhyme, and storytelling techniques. In African-American cultures, then, retention of the spoken word (memory) is depended upon more often and face-to-face communication is frequent and highly valued. In contrast, those living in the United States assume, for the most part, that if something is in print then it is true. The written word is viewed as having more value and is therefore more credible. What this shows for the two groups just mentioned is that if the written or spoken message is in symbols acceptable to the receiver and uses his most acceptable channels, then it will be more understandable. A combination of channels is often the most helpful. If an activity is demonstrated or diagrammed, explained verbally with the aid of written instruction, the receiver may feel more secure that he understands the message. The sender, also, may rest assured that a diverse audience can be reached; it comprehends the message via the individual receiver's most used channels. In establishing initial contact, it is more important to know which channels to use and which sources are most credible to those we wish to reach.

The message communicated is organized around language. There is one special communication concept, the Whorfian Principle, which states that language determines, organizes, and limits thought. The number of words an Arctic dweller has for "snow," or the words an American uses in place of "automobile" give some indication of the central nature of these concepts within regional thought and communication. Even when a language is shared there are regional nuances, slang, professional jargon, teenage "in" words, and colloquialisms. Individually valued or emotionally laden words also may confuse, facilitate, or block communication.

Emotionally laden words or values attached to given words may serve as barriers to understanding or accepting communication: the use of obscenity, for example, or when what is communicated is inconsistent with or contrary to the receiver's values or preferences. For the person who has just had a stroke and is expecting full recovery, instructions on adapting to disability may well fall on deaf ears. When overwhelming loss occurs, a common experience among the elderly, denial of sad realities is often the first reaction: any communication that attempts to confront or deal with the loss is blocked. Thus instruction, facts, even caring intentions may be initially rejected. They may be integrated later when the person is at a stage of acceptance. It is important to observe responses and listen to questions; they often indicate what the elderly person is ready to hear.

CROSS-CULTURAL CONCEPTS:
COMMUNICATION ACROSS GENERATIONS

The nonverbal component of the message conveyed is most important. Depending upon which expert one consults, the nonverbal aspect of communication comprises from 55 to 97 percent of the message. Nonverbal communication supports or negates the spoken word. The concepts we shall discuss here include kinesics (body language), homophile, proxemics (space), time, and touch. Rules and values are attached to nonverbal interactions and they vary greatly in cultural usage.

Kinesics, a term coined by Birdwhistle, relates to body language, posture, body positioning, facial expressions, and interaction rituals. These rituals occur in our daily relations with others and are composed of varying sequences that may signify courting, mating, greeting, farewell, and other communication intentions. In cross-cultural communication, it has been noted that each language has a concommitant nonverbal pattern of gestures. These are concurrently communicated with the spoken language. Thus, if both verbalization and nonverbal patterns are simultaneous and congruent, the message is credible. If, however, one speaks French but gestures in English, the message is confusing and its clarity leaves something to be desired.

The most significant form of nonverbal communication is eye contact. Through eye contact we recognize the existence of those individuals around us: we indicate that a person may speak, is being listened to, or grant permission to enter a group. A teacher may pressure a student into compliance with little more than the strategic use of a prolonged stare. Seductive interactions are accomplished with the perfectly timed glance. In North American culture, honesty is equated with direct eye contact. The honest man "looks you straight in the eye," while the liar may be described as shifty-eyed or as one who can't or won't look others in the eye when speaking. On the other hand, persons can be ignored or their existence denied by not looking in their direction. Exclusion from a group can be accomplished by lack of eye contact from individuals within the group.

Listening and attending behaviors are also reinforced through eye contact and body positioning. Leaning toward another, tilting one's head, crossing one's legs in the direction of another usually indicates awareness and openness toward that person. In groups, people are made to feel included through body positioning, eye contact, and gestures. In a group of three, body language may indicate which two are the couple, who is informing whom, or who the leader is by the person's vigorous motion and intensity as well as his timing of eye contact and response. Preferences, liaisons, and relationships may be communicated with body language and eye contact.

In like manner, folded arms, turning one's back on another, leaning back or away, and putting one's feet up may communicate rejection, unwillingness to listen, or a closed mind.

Schefelen has written an entire book documenting a one-hour psycho-analytic session between a female patient, her mother, the psychoanalyst, and a psychiatric resident. This analysis traces the verbalizations along with the simultaneous nonverbal behaviors that occur. The nonverbal patterns indicated binding and resistive behaviors, agreement and liaisons, intrusions, and directions taken during this therapeutic hour. A glance toward another may indicate such messages as agreement, inclusion, or the granting of permission to speak. A glance away may communicate disagreement; rejection of the person, his statement, or both; exclusion; or denial.

Interaction rituals include a specific sequence of well-timed behaviors, words, and actions appropriate to role, along with occasion and level of relationship and interaction. Examples include greetings, farewells, courtships, celebrations, as well as everyday work rituals and behaviors. These rituals vary among nations, cultures, sexes, age groups, and even from family to family. Businessmen may meet, quickly look one another in the eye, shake hands, then sit down to lunch. Determining which individuals exhibit leadership behaviors will depend upon dominance, territoriality, and communication skills as well as roles and relationships. Specific contexts of interaction and the rules of each particular group will assist in determining such social customs as the appropriate length of time to wait for someone, who is to extend his hand first in greeting, the length of eye contact, whether one or both parties look down, whether looking down is an indication of respect or submission, and a whole host of other rituals.

Thus, in the interaction ritual of greeting, names and titles are voiced, endearments or introductions extended, heads nod, hands may be shaken, embraces exchanged, and directions given. Who addresses whom, with what formal titles or informal words or touch, and how individuals present themselves to one another are components considered in this sequential interaction. In an initial interaction with an older person, the preferred name and title should be elicited and used to indicate respect for the individuality of the person. Establishing the correct or most comfortable form of address, including spelling and pronunciation, is one way to recognize each person as both unique and worthwhile. Use of the first name, especially when permission has not been given, could be demeaning and may in fact communicate a lack of concern or respect for the older person. Taking a few minutes to explain who you are and how your role or position relates to the individual's needs or interests can prove to be an invaluable first step when interacting with older persons:

Mr. Brown, I'm Dr. Gross, the occupational therapist who will be working with you each morning from 9 to 10. We'll be working together to evaluate your daily activity schedule. We'll be setting goals and priorities and planning for any adjustments that might need to be made before you return home and resume work.

Soliciting input and ideas to obtain participation in communicating goals, feelings, and suggestions is important at the outset if good rapport is to be established in the communication interaction. The first interaction is crucial and often sets the tone of attitudes and expectations:

"He doesn't listen to me or hear; he just tells me what to do, when he doesn't even know what I can do."

"She always notices how I look and remembers what I like to do and my goals and ideas."

"I wish my grandson treated me like you do!"

Positive expectations based on the initial interaction usually promote future cooperation and participation.

Proxemics, or space as it affects human communication across cultures, can be examined in three contexts: (1) interpersonal space as it defines and establishes the depth and level of intimacy in communication; (2) organization of space, which determines the type or content of communication activity; and (3) space as territoriality, examined by Ardrey in *Territorial Imperative* and Lorenz in *On Aggression*. They describe the group behaviors, mating rituals, and the establishment of territoriality in animals as a basis for understanding human communication behaviors.

Hall describes four levels of personal space that relate to human interpersonal communication. The first, called the *intimate level,* is from personal contact to one foot of distance. This would include parent-child communication and intimate relations. Personal communication on a regular basis, occurring between persons on an intense interactional level, occurs at a distance of between one and three feet. This is the average American's personal space, the *comfort level,* that thirty-six-inch perimeter forming the most common and acceptable boundary at which one-to-one communication occurs. The third level of social interaction generally occurs within a three- to twelve-foot boundary. This is often exemplified in the organization and arrangement of a typical American *living room* where chairs, sofas, coffee tables, and end tables are placed at a distance comfortable for socializing. The last level, *public space,* is defined by Hall as anything beyond twelve feet. Interactions in a school or church setting and addressing political rallies or public gatherings would be examples of public forms of communication.

The personal space that defines communication varies across cultures, with people from populous countries and urban cultures, including Oriental and South American peoples, needing and using less space. Americans typically have a three-foot personal space boundary, whereas others may more comfortably communicate within an eighteen-inch perimeter. Sommers, in *Personal Space,* describes the schizophrenic person as one who is unable to recognize appropriate personal space rules for communication, and either intrudes on another's boundaries or maintains too great a distance. When more space is needed but not readily available, as is the case in many cities, individuals may protect themselves or establish individual space by reading a paper or magazine, positioning their bodies in carefully orchestrated ways to lay claim to space, avoiding eye contact when entering a crowded elevator, or by placing physical dividers.

Work space is similarly organized in a manner conducive to work requirements and the amount of communication preferred or required. Managers, counselors, and others who spend the major portion of their workday in interpersonal communication have space arranged for control of interactions. Chairs, desks, and other objects are positioned at appropriate distances to maintain eye contact. Distractions and intrusions are eliminated and arrangements are kept flexible enough for one-to-one or group communication.

Territoriality is a third communication concept related to our use of space. A typical health-care professional provides care within a hospital or clinic. This territory is familiar, secure, and controlled by the caregiver. When in home health care, however, the setting is owned by and familiar to the client; the caregiver then gains entry and provides help on the other's turf after first obtaining permission. In public or neutral settings, the determination of who owns or provides the territory relates to who has control of the communication event.

The older person within the health care system will be on unfamiliar territory and will find professional jargon and the language relating to illness both confusing and unsettling. Medical terminology is of necessity used to describe and define, and care is for the most part provided by persons much younger and from different backgrounds than their older clients. Familiar settings and recognizable symbols, language, and events offer security and are conducive to more and better communication. Often the elderly person, who functions well at home and in a familiar community, will become confused and disoriented when hospitalized or placed in a new and strange setting.

The concept of time is interpreted very differently in the United States than it is in African, South American, or Asian cultures. We value time, using it as a unit of measure to determine intelligence, comprehension, and even performance. This timing of daily functions often places the older citizen at a disadvantage since there may be some physical or mental slowing of motor, sensory, or cognitive faculties. Appearing a few minutes late for an appointment or completing a task later than others may result in the person being characterized as irresponsible, uncooperative, disorganized, or lazy. If the person happens to be elderly, additional attributes are affixed such as forgetful, senile, or exhibiting symptoms of Alzheimer's disease.

Americans also use time as a framework for structuring interactions and, indeed, our daily schedules. Our allocation of time reflects our priorities. Americans and the English are always scheduling, whereas in most other cultures the unit of value is the task to be accomplished. Meetings must begin and end on schedule for the American businessperson traveling overseas. Interactions are planned in order to catch the 5 o'clock plane or for the next scheduled appointment. In other cultures, it may be considered rude to set and follow a precisely-timed schedule. Of primary importance is the interaction or the relationship. Thus, sufficient time and attention are devoted to an interaction until it is satisfactorily accomplished. This approach is generally the most valued in the rest of the world. To Americans, time is spent or wasted since "time is money, time is precious." Physicians, typically, will schedule many patients at the same time, ensuring that most will be kept waiting, causing delays and inconvenience. Keeping others waiting may be one example of showing or communicating higher status. In other words, the one who keeps others waiting is reflecting the fact that he or she possesses higher status and has more control than one who waits. The elderly are often kept waiting. In academic settings, students have been expected to wait five minutes for a tardy instructor, ten minutes for an assistant professor, fifteen for an associate professor, and twenty for the full professor who is late!

Human touch may communicate warmth, love, oneness and support or it may be perceived as an invasion of privacy. Touch can be depersonalizing when a health-care provider pokes, probes, explores an individual without obtaining permission, explaining the purpose, or discussing the results. This type of invasive touch ignores the person and communicates that what is being examined is a "thing," a "disease," or "an interesting case." It can be demeaning or frightening to the individual being examined. Often, in addition to the impersonal use of touch, discussion of the person's condition excludes the patient entirely. Touch, in another negative sense, may be used to dominate or direct communication. The health-care professional touches the patient, but the patient is prevented from reaching out and touching in return. Many dominant-submissive relationships are reflected by who touches whom and in what context. For example, a supervisor may walk up behind a secretary and observe work from behind while remaining unobserved, or touch the secretary's shoulder while the latter is seated and at a disadvantage. All these are examples of a dominant position.

Touch can reassure and communicate friendship and caring. When a person is hospitalized in an unfamiliar setting with unfamiliar objects and people, the hug of a friend or the touch of a hand may be most supportive. One physician, after daily rounds were completed late in the evening, would enter a dying patient's room and sit, holding the person's hand for a prolonged period of time. This conveyed an important message: "I care, I'm here for you, and I'm ready to listen or just to be with you." For the person who has suffered the loss of a significant other, status, or health, the physical contact of a hug or a touch can be the much-needed link to life and meaning. Often touch may be comforting when words are difficult to find and/or express.

The establishment of a common base of shared meaning and experience is vital when initiating communication. We tend to be mutually attracted, to agree with and understand, those we see as most similar to ourselves. Thus, if another looks similar; expresses the same opinions or beliefs; or attends the same school, church, or synagogue the assumption is that he will also share our attitudes and values. One is apt to marry the boy or girl next door because of proximity and shared life experiences. Contrary to popular myth, likes do attract. Mutuality provides comfort and communicates a basis for both understanding and empathy. An older person may feel safer and in better hands if it is known that the younger health professional is from the same region, has parents who belong to the same church or club, or is interested in the same sports team. In actual collaboration with the elderly, establishing common goals, priorities, and concerns also indicates respect for the person's ideas, engages active participation, and contributes to patient receptivity.

Credibility, or belief in the source of communication, is also facilitated by the establishment of a common base of beliefs, attitudes, and values. We tend to believe and hear those persons we consider to be most in accord with our beliefs, attitudes, values, and past experiences. In addition, if two people originally agree, the expectation is established that there will be further areas of agreement. When communication begins with disagreement or misunderstanding, on the other hand, the care provider may be considered neither caring nor a credible source of factual information.

Peers, because it is assumed that they are coming from the same place and have shared the same hopes, fears, and life experiences, are usually considered credible sources. One may consult one's colleague, a student in the same class, or a patient in the same room to obtain and share information. The supervisor, teacher, or nurse may have the information needed and be more accurate but might not be considered as approachable or as understanding. Working with the elderly in groups often enlists and enables them to help and support one another since the peer group will be perceived as less threatening.

Another major category of credible sources includes those viewed as experts or leaders in a given community. Initially, our most credible sources were parents and family members who shaped our beliefs and values. As life progresses, teachers become important sources of information. Peers enter to test or modify our beliefs and attitudes. Other major credible sources include clergy, community and political leaders, physicians, counselors, and others considered to be experts who are consulted and believed to be helpful. People in one's own age group are considered credible because of similar or shared life experiences, as are those who are older because of the extent and breadth of their experience.

Since information given is based upon the speaker's background, experiences, and beliefs, and this information perceived by another's set of beliefs, attitudes, and values, there is great potential for misinformation or misperception. If one who likes fish is asked to recommend the best restaurant, the recommendation may be inappropriate to one who does not appreciate seafood. Clarity and feedback are important concepts here. The question must be clarified in order to give the appropriate answer.

Symbolic communication that occurs through the choice of dress, objects, and activities is important to observe and also to interpret. The older person's dress may reflect freedom of choice, creativity, lifestyle, self-concept, or intended purposes. Institutional or impersonal clothes may indicate status as a patient or loss of life roles and control over decision making. Roles and personality are often reflected via dress. When this choice is eliminated or prohibited, it diminishes individuality and serves to depersonalize. The therapist may provide formality, security, or comfort by wearing a uniform; a more human image is conveyed when both client and professional are individually dressed.

Name tags, professional emblems, and uniform garb serve to indicate roles and status and thus establish expectations in an interaction. Often the person in white is immediately seen as one who can help someone in distress or pain, while to a child it may be the one who inflicts pain with a needle. To the confused person, it can be reassuring to identify a helper by name tag and/or dress.

Transitional objects that people carry from one stage of life or place to another may include pictures, books, and gifts received on important occasions from significant others. These objects may have great meaning and can provide considerable security in a new, threatening, or confusing situation. Encouraging the elderly to take their own furniture, clothes, plants, pictures, and other objects into a new living space may make it more their own and less confusing or depersonalizing. Nursing homes that encourage residents to bring their own furnishings decrease the disorientation felt in a new setting. Pets may provide opportunities to nurture, care for, and touch another living thing. The lack of familiar objects within one's lifespace may increase disengagement, thus decreasing meaning in life as well as undermining any feeling the elderly might have of being needed.

The kinds and extent of participation in activities may communicate one's self-concept, self-confidence, feelings regarding competence, and one's ability to perform. In like manner, activities that are provided or suggested to elderly persons reflect the communicator's perception of the older person's abilities and potential. Objects or activities engaged in may serve as gifts and express love, care, and continuity of a relationship. They also may provide those who participate with an opportunity for choice, enjoyment, and some control and verification in their daily functioning. When a caregiver takes an object away, repeats or modifies it, it is no longer a reflection of personal or individual ability.

Engaging in activity provides an opportunity to observe and evaluate the self-concept as communicated by rules taken, decisions made or deferred, and the quality of the product or activity outcome. Whether a person resists, is hesitant, or eagerly seeks out activities also communicates something about her attitudes and approach to life, her general health, and her willingness to engage with others. Withdrawal from activities, asocial behavior, or detachment from others may reflect a perfectly normal approach to life, signify depression, or indicate individual personality preferences. The manner in which activities are organized and carried out are often determined by life roles, culturally-determined rules, and self-perception of competence as exhibited in performance.

COMMUNICATION PRINCIPLES: BASICS AND EXAMPLES

Turning again to the human components in the communication model, the sender and the receiver, the focus of communication is what goes on inside and between the participants while they are engaged in dealing with task activity, verbal and nonverbal content, and feedback. Communication between two people is constantly in flux, depending upon perceptions, feedback, and interpretation by each individual. Indeed, it is amazing, all factors considered, that communication so often does occur—that meaning is shared.

Some basic communication principles broadly apply in facilitating this sharing:

1. It is more confirming to be recognized as existing than to be treated as nonexisting. Using the addressed person's correct title, calling the person by a preferred name, and remembering special concerns of the other indicate that the person's existence is important. Eye contact; physical contact via a hug, handshake, or gentle touch; and special questions directed to the other facilitate interaction. In essence, these techniques say, "You're important—your thoughts, feelings and opinions are important to me." Asking questions that indicate respect for the aged person's expertise and interests, and eliciting their involvement by seeking opinions, ideas, and participation show that the person addressed is valued. "What would be your favorite birthday dinner?" "What kind of apple trees did you raise; which are the best?" "How did you find Paris when you visited after twenty years?" "What do you like to grow in your garden?" are examples of open, easy-to-answer questions. These questions elicit feelings, opinions, likes and dislikes based on past positive experiences. This type of question also relates to an individual's positive contributions in the here and now. Asking for or requiring the aged person's input into treatment planning, priority setting, or retirement planning recognizes the individual's centrality while involving her participation from the outset.

   In contrast, talking in front of, beyond, through, or about another person without eye contact, touch, or inclusion is an all too frequent occurence. It is depersonalizing. The individual may not be included in plans or decisions concerning her life: she is discussed as a thing, a problem, a case, or a confused child unable to control her personal environment. Body language—such as turning one's back or similar inattentive body positioning—can also deny another's importance or existence.

2. Dialogue is more confirming than monologue. Lectures, sermons, and other one-way directives limit or prevent active participation and feedback. When the patient is not allowed to question, clarify, or expand upon information provided, instructions may not be understood or applied. Health-care personnel who use medical terminology when giving instructions may not be fully understood. Instructions cannot be followed when the patient wonders about the how, the why, or the when of medication or therapeutic exercises. One-way communication is often authoritarian and noninclusive; whereas the more dialogue there is, the more meaning is shared.

3. Acceptance is more confirming than interpretation. An attitude of acceptance of the individual will provide a strong basis on which to develop rapport and trust. Indeed, it is a prerequisite for developing an empathic, facilitative interaction. Showing respect for another's ideas and opinions, listening without argument or interruption, and reflecting back to clarify not only indicate understanding but also communicate acceptance. Interpretation before the communicator has an opportunity to state or explain her meaning communicates impatience as well as lack of acceptance. "Oh yes, I know what you mean, but it won't work here," is one such example. When interpretation is done prior to acceptance, there will be little basis for mutual understanding.

4. It is more confirming to be treated personally than impersonally. Recognizing individual preferences, observing personal space, using eye contact, and incorporating individual name and form of address are examples that show recognition of the person as an individual.

In one nursing text, a multitude of two-sentence examples were given to recognize the individual patient in a healthy, normal human manner. The first sentence addressed the person by title and name, then made an observation concerning something noted about the patient that had nothing to do with being a sick person (a patient). The second sentence asked a question related to the first factual observation. Examples might be, "Mrs. Green, that nail polish is a lovely new color. What is it called?" Or, "Dr. Johnson, you had your hair cut and styled since I saw you this morning. Who cut and styled it for you?" In addition to recognizing the individual person, it is communicated that healthy, normal behaviors are seen and expected. Too often with the elderly only comments and questions concerning problems, illness, or infirmity are introduced. Discussion then remains centered upon negatives and interaction may be dreaded by either party. Personhood may be fragmented by comments that relate only to disabling problems. The whole person, including positive performance and ideas, is not allowed to emerge or participate.

5. Openness—sharing of feelings, observations, and experiences—can promote mutuality, a feeling of working together and sharing. It may be important for the elderly to share here-and-now feelings and their reasons, especially when caregivers may be upset, have a bad day, or be negatively affected by outside or personal issues. The older person may feel rejected or concerned that the caregiver's

anger is directed toward him/her. "I got up late, my car wouldn't start, my son was ill, and the baby sitter's on vacation!" would serve to clarify that the elderly person isn't the cause or the target of impatience or anger. Sharing joy and enthusiasm can also promote more conversational give-and-take. "Our team won!" "Let's celebrate; I won the lottery!" "I love those roses, they're my favorite kind and color!" Expressing individual opinions may equalize communication and sharing. Showing enthusiasm for an activity or an idea can facilitate further participation. Noting individual things shows appreciation for an individual: "You wear various shades of pink so well—is it your favorite color?" "Your flowers bloom continually from early spring through the fall. Did you plan the seasonal blooms and color combinations you have?"

6. A here-and-now orientation is vital for facilitating focusing, controlling, and living in the present. This is especially true with the aged who may have less positive present experiences. They tend to withdraw to more pleasant past experiences and behaviors. Focusing on interests, healthy activities, and decisions concerning today's schedule, where the aged person has some control and choice, is important. Asking questions pertaining to past skills that could transfer well into the present cultivates participation and appreciation for the present. This also allows, recognizes, and commends application of expertise, interests, and skills in the present. "I understand you've always sewn your clothes and are quite skillful. I seem to have hit a snag and need help with my machine. Would you be willing to take a look at it?" "A number of the clubwomen are interested in quilting and I hear you're the expert. Would you be willing to teach a class or help me set one up?" "I understand you're the organic gardener on your block. Do you make your own compost?"

7. Spontaneity is another quality that allows more creativity and flexibility in interaction. It makes change easier to implement and less frightening at times. It also can make for a more open, accepting, comfortable, and participative atmosphere. Expressing feelings openly as they occur or asking for help and obtaining ideas can promote more cooperative communication. Listening, remembering, and following through on spontaneous suggestions offered by the elderly will encourage further contributions on their part. "Mr. Winston, when we were planning Saturday's schedule you mentioned a special function at the Arboretum. It seems a good day for a

walk there—what do you think?" "Sam, you mentioned being hungry for cheesecake, and Mrs. Jefferson makes the best, I hear. Shall we encourage her to try one on us?"

Other forms of facilitative communication include authenticity, self-disclosure, and trust. Unhelpful responses can include interruptions, irrelevancies, and incongruous conversations.

ESTABLISHING A SUPPORTIVE
CLIMATE FOR COMMUNICATION

Developing a healthy, supportive communication climate will provide a firm base of rapport, trust, and empathy upon which in-depth, helpful, and ongoing communication can be established. Facilitating a supportive attitude and approach can be promoted if one bears in mind the following concepts of helpful versus unhelpful approaches:

1. Use descriptive rather than evaluative speech. Thus, instead of evaluating a person as one who "is hostile, uncooperative, and refuses to do anything," describing the actual behavior and words may be more accurate, objective, and helpful. An example of the latter is, "He said he'd had a bad weekend, was tired and coming down with the flu. Also, he'd never liked carpentry. He then returned to his room." Even positive evaluative statements may be perceived as judgmental and thus limit interaction. "That's great!" or "That's right," when a person may have meant to ask for help or clarification can stifle further questions, especially if one is having difficulty or wishes to make a suggestion.

2. Using a problem-solving approach rather than maintaining control can facilitate more equal give-and-take as well as participation. If the sender needs to direct or control, "you should . . ." or "have to . . ." communication will tend to be one-way with little opportunity for feedback. If an approach of "Let's sit down and see what we can come up with" is used, a contract is possible, one in which goals and priorities are established together. Decisions then can be made and implemented.

3. A spontaneous atmosphere with freedom to express feelings, needs, and ideas promotes more interaction than when there have been closely planned strategies to control a meeting. A tightly timed

schedule can defeat the purpose of an interaction if time is the main unit determining the process of a meeting. Americans often make this error in international meetings and discussions, maintaining such rigid and precise timing that greater interactional priorities are forgotten. An inflexible, predetermined agenda can also contribute to feelings of entrapment wherein there is no opportunity to contribute items or review the agenda of a meeting prior to discussion. Asking for input when most decisions have already been made also decreases further contributions.

4. Empathy, the ability to put oneself in another's position and feel what another is experiencing, communicates an attitude of understanding and desire to communicate. Asking for feedback to better understand the interests, goals, directions, and feelings of the receiver facilitates two-way communication and contribution. Contrariwise, an attitude of neutrality, often hidden behind objectivity, may communicate a lack of concern and involvement. Expressing warmth and enthusiasm can be supportive as opposed to maintaining neutrality or distancing oneself from the elderly person.

5. Projecting an attitude of equality versus one of superiority is usually more facilitative. The elderly, those who are depressed, or those who prefer to have others make their decisions for them will be relieved initially, perhaps, to be told what to do. This will not serve, however, to gain their participation later. Planning and working collaboratively and cooperatively promotes mutual respect and opportunities for more input and flexibility in further contributions.

6. A provisional "Let's give it a try—it's not etched in concrete" approach is more conducive to ongoing communication than an attitude of certainty: "There's only one right way to do this." A temporary solution usually is more acceptable.

COMMUNICATION BARRIERS

There are any number of reasons two people may not be able to share meaning. As previously mentioned, if the initial interaction is one of disagreement or establishes differences or a lack of commonality, then establishing ongoing communication may be difficult. Barriers may be present in either party initially or may develop from negative feedback as communication continues.

When a person is angry, preoccupied, upset, or in crisis there may be difficulty in hearing, understanding, and/or focusing. The receiver's ability to see, hear, or participate will be impaired by her inward focus. Energy and perception cannot be directed outward when there is inward preoccupation. For example, when a person has just been diagnosed as having cancer, it may be impossible to hear any further communication concerning implication, good news, or self-help instructions. When one is angry at another, his/her intentions and suggestions will be under suspicion; the other person will not be seen as helpful, and his/her comments may be misconstrued because of the cloud of anger blocking perceptions.

When the message is confused or unclear because of problems with words or nonverbal contradictions presented by the speaker, communication may be blocked. However, if the receiver is able to reflect back and provide feedback on what was heard, or if the receiver can question the speaker to clarify meaning, it may enable the speaker to clarify or modify the message, putting it into a more understandable form.

Precipitous, superficial interpretation before a message is completed can impede open communication. Examples are "I see," or "Oh, you obviously have a communication problem. What you should do. . . ." Trite, quick, impatient statements that oversimplify what the person is saying can communicate unwillingness to listen or a lack of concern for the speaker. In like manner, advice extended before the problems are clarified or before a mutual contract for working together is established may be neither helpful nor welcome.

Distractions, in the form of interruptions, noise, or multichannel input can fragment, overwhelm, or irritate. In an interview, for instance, time should be planned so it is convenient for participants and adequate for the interaction. Telephone, visual, and personnel interruptions should be eliminated or minimized. The interview area should be distraction-free. The space should be arranged to facilitate interaction so the right space and eye contact can be maintained. Objects in view should be relevant to the situation and not extraneous clutter.

Multiple sensory input can be confusing to anyone. For the elderly, sorting out varied simultaneous sensory input can be both difficult and tiring. Sounds may ring in one's ears and information can be difficult to organize, select from, and make into a sensible whole. Decreasing sensory stimulation, whether it be auditory, visual, or olfactory in nature, may be needed in order to focus and communicate successfully with an elderly person. If there is background music, it should be familiar and relaxing, not stimulating or jarring. Speaking slowly and clearly, using familiar examples and terminology, and focusing on the person may decrease confusion and irritation caused by multiple stimuli. Familiar words, sounds, and visual symbols related to the interaction could facilitate listening and communication.

Hearing problems are the most common block to communicating with the elderly on a sensory level. The hard-of-hearing individual will miss even more of what is being communicated when there is no eye contact. Thus, facing the person so visual cues such as lip reading and gestures can be observed will compensate to a certain degree. Using a low tone of voice when speaking is usually the easiest to hear since hearing loss most often occurs in the higher registers. Unfortunately, many people attempt to communicate with the hard-of-hearing by standing over them and shouting in a loud or raised tone of voice. Hearing deprivation can be frightening also, and cause further problems. Initial footsteps or comments of those entering an area are missed and the hearing-impaired person is startled or jarred when someone comes up quickly without the relied-upon auditory warning. Thus, keeping within the receiver's visual as well as tonal range aids communication. When this is not observed, responses from the hearing-impaired person may be suspicious, irritable, angry, or disoriented in nature. When others are laughing or talking and glances are turned toward someone outside the group, the communication to the hearing-impaired may be, "We're talking about and laughing at you." Resistance to wearing a hearing aid is often occasioned by ill-fitting, poorly-adjusted devices and may be interpreted by helpers as rigidity or resistance. Cosmetic aspects as well as discomfort may make the hard-of-hearing person loath to use the hearing aid. Obtaining the aid may prove a financial hardship. Moreover, devices or surgery do not correct all hearing impairments.

Depression is a common problem with the retired person. Indeed, the suicide rate in the elderly is considerably higher than statistics would indicate. Death from malnutrition and alcoholism may be further evidence of depressive behaviors. Many healthy persons, whatever their age, when suffering loss of status, vocation, family, friends, or colleagues can undergo depressive episodes. These episodes occur more often and may be simultaneous in the elderly person. The resulting natural grief reaction needs to be identified so that the grieving process can be undergone and facilitated. At times, however, multiple losses of significant others may be overwhelming, causing immobilization, withdrawal, and/or depression.

Depression is exhibited in varying ways, including slowed speech, motor movement, and verbal responses; cognitive and motor retardation; slowed thought processing and responses due to sadness, inner focus, and preoccupation. Depression will be a barrier to communication and will require specific methods and approaches in order to share meaning and interact with the person undergoing a depressive episode. The depressed person, then, has difficulty paying attention, focusing, listening, and making choices and decisions. The person may be mute or appear nonresponsive, rejecting, or agitated. It may not be possible to obtain eye contact, verbal response, or action upon instruction from the depressed person. A common appearance is that of dejection—looking down or moving slowly if at all—with verbalization limited to monosyllables, phrases, apologies, or physical manifestations of anxiety.

Perception of the depressed person, because of the withdrawal and lack of response, may be that of someone who is uncooperative, resistive, sick, deteriorating, or suffering from organic brain disease or trauma. Competency and intelligence tests may be lowered because of this depressive overlay. A lack of interest, concern, or affect may be communicated. Diagnoses or perceptions of the person exhibiting depressive behaviors can lead to further negative misinterpretation, hampering communication even after the depression has lifted. Thus negative labeling of an elderly person is sometimes initiated when the individual is undergoing a depressive reaction. This may affect further performance expectations.

Sensory loss or deterioration may diminish, retard, or stop communication. Hearing loss impedes communication processes as well as affecting attitudes, perceptions, and self-image. Visual loss or dimunition also slows information input, lessens clarity, and will be a special barrier to those most dependent upon the written word, diagrams, or demonstrations. Communication is most effective when multiple sensory channels are used. When several senses are dimmed, such as smell, hearing, sight, and touch, communication clarity/intensity/meaning may well be lessened. There may be gaps and missing connections, and these may lead to misunderstanding and feelings of confusion.

A poor self-concept may be a barrier to communication. If the sender of a message feels uncertain, insecure, or devalued, her communication may also lack confidence, clarity, and strength. The older American nearing retirement may be dealing with multiple losses: status, job, financial security, and colleagues. The perception of self as in control of one's life, as provider for others with potential for further growth and success may be lost. The external perception of the retired individual as communicated by others is often that of one who possesses limited power, diminished potential, and reduced participation ability. The older worker may be ignored in planning and decision-making functions at work. He or she may no longer be consulted by spouse, children, and neighbors. Thus, their perceptions of themselves as worthwhile, important, contributing members of society are diminished both internally and externally.

Role transitions or reversals may cause anger, confusion, and resistance when communicating with the elderly whose physical, mental, and/or financial status is diminishing. The provider, decision-maker, the head-of-family upon whom others were dependent may retire or become ill and dependent. Being able to ask others for help, accept help from others, and being dependent upon others may be frightening, unacceptable, confusing, and depressing. Others affected in the relationship may find themselves in reversed roles. They also may feel confused, angry, and unable to cope. Feelings and competencies associated with lifelong roles are threatened and overturned. When a very stable pattern of communication is completely reversed, the meanings, roles, perceptions, and symbols are no longer familiar. Expectations, then, are not met in relationships. Establishing communication regarding these transitions in roles, and the meaning and implications to those involved, is crucial to understanding and accepting new models and roles.

Catastrophic illness such as a heart attack, stroke, or accident injury may immediately immobilize a person and alter feelings of self-worth as well as views about one's ability to contribute, provide, and participate. The former provider is now the one being provided for. The mutual husband-wife team who discussed life-goals and made decisions now has one passive partner who may not be able to speak. The ability to ask for help or hear suggestions may be blocked by the impact of the crisis.

Myths and fallacies concerning the aging abound. These affect expectations relating to competency in performance and when voiced by colleagues, family, and friends, often affect self-esteem. Some of these fallacies, so often voiced, become integrated and believed by the elderly persons themselves, thus resulting in self-fulfilling prophesies. Some common myths that create barriers to participation or demean the elderly include:

1. Most elderly people are sick, incapacitated, and end up in nursing homes. The fact is that the majority of elderly people are healthy. Only 5 percent are in nursing homes. Unfortunately, these myths do affect expectations; retired persons do make more doctors' appointments, which may be indicative of sharing society's expectation that retirement and ill health are correlated.

2. The fallacy that the older person can't learn and that mental capacities diminish is often voiced, as in "You can't teach an old dog new tricks!" On the contrary, many elderly not only take up where they left off with past interests and relationships, but many learn new skills; graduate from college; or begin aerobics, music lessons, traveling, new jobs or avocations.

3. Comments pertaining to living in the past and senility relate to only a few older persons. Discussing past memories and experiences is,

moreover, an important life task. Positive life contributions and experiences from the past may be more pleasant reference points than present problems and diminishing interactions. These successful past experiences may be referred to or brought into the present in an effort to maintain hope and self-esteem.

4. The perception of the elderly as needy or in need is often projected. This assumption generalizes the older population as unidimensional—poor, dependent, sick, and needing assistance. Their ability to contribute, provide, consult, advise, or enable others is denied by the artificial barrier of age, even though it has little or nothing to do with actual competence or performance.

5. The expectation that older people can't or don't contribute erects an artificial barrier to their participation. Activities of the Gray Panthers, the American Association of Retired Persons, as well as many other groups of older persons have greatly contributed to legislation, conservation, and change in society. In *Old, Poor, Alone and Happy: How to Live Nicely on Practically Nothing,* the author—a retired woman named Katherine Dissinger—discusses myriad ways of coping with poverty, dealing with life transitions, establishing new goals and priorities, and contributing to younger people in their areas of need. Volunteers, many of whom are older Americans, contribute energy, ideas, and hours of devoted service to many helping agencies.

SUMMARY: COMMUNICATION WITH THE ELDERLY

In review, to facilitate shared meaning those who work with the elderly should focus on the most facilitative channels, familiar language, and nonverbal components of the message while bearing in mind the individual receiver's perceptions, interpretations, and feedback. Some critical concepts to observe in communicating with the elderly, as well as others, would thus include some of the following precepts:

1. Initially establish a common bond of agreement on beliefs, attitudes, values, or priorities. This initial mutual agreement establishes the expectations of further mutual agreement. Identification of common background experiences, interests, and affiliations provides a feeling of security or familiarity with the older person.

2. Communicate to the healthy person that skills, interests, and abilities are recognized and valued. Include the total person rather than focusing only on problems.

3. Recognize the unique individual: remember correct names and titles. Include past interests and contributed ideas so that communication is personalized.

4. Establish a mutually-participative communication where goals and priorities are discussed and decided upon together, and where each person has a role in their implementation. Expect that the older person will contribute a wealth of ideas and skills.

5. Use humor when appropriate, especially if the older person shares an appreciation of certain forms of humor—jokes, poems, ditties, cartoons.

6. Determine the most facilitative channel or combination of channels. Language and symbols need to be familiar and conducive to communication. Determine which factors are particular barriers in communicating with the individual.

7. Observe special cultural, financial, physical, emotional, cognitive, or social changes the person is experiencing; these may reduce ability to communicate.

8. Be sensitive to indications of reaction to loss, grief, and depression, all of which need to be identified and expressed.

9. Be aware of specific sensory problems that may impede communication.

A vast expanse of life experiences and transitions have already been enjoyed or experienced by many elderly people. The more understanding and skill we can bring into our communication across generations and cultures, the closer we will come to sharing meaning in a mutually satisfying manner.

FOR DISCUSSION

1. Suggest five areas of commonality to engage an elderly neighbor in drawing on past areas of expertise in an initial meeting.

2. Identify five comments and/or phrases in daily conversation that serve to devalue or demean the elderly person.
3. State three facts about the elderly that discount commonly voiced negative stereotypes and assumptions.
4. State three examples of organizations working for the elderly, either local, regional, or national.
5. Phrase three opening statements that would set healthy, mutually participative expectations in communicating with an elderly person.

BIBLIOGRPAHY

American Occupational Therapy Association. *The Role of Occupational Therapy with the Elderly.* Rockville, Md.: American Occupational Therapy Association, 1985

Berlo, David. *The Process of Communication,* New York: Holt, Rinehart and Winston, Inc., 1968.

Burnside, Irene (ed.). *Working with the Elderly: Group Process and Techniques.* Monterey, Calif.: Wadsworth, Inc., 1984

Gross, Dellvina. "Therapeutic Communication," Eighth International Congress, World Federation of Occupational Therapists, Vol. I, 1982.

Hall, Edwin T. *The Hidden Dimension.* New York: Doubleday & Dell, 1966

———. *Beyond Culture.* New York: Anchor Press, 1976.

Lewis, Sandra Cutler. *Providing for the Older Adult: A Gerontological Handbook.* Thorofare, N.J.: Slack, Inc., 1983.

Schlossberg, Nancy K. *Counseling Adults in Transition: Linking Practice with Theory.* New York: Springer Publishing Company, 1984.

Sommers, Robert. *Personal Space: The Behavioral Basis of Design.* Englewood Cliffs, N.J.: Prentice-Hall, Inc., 1969.

Stewart, E. C. *American Cultural Patterns: A Crosscultural Perspective.* Pittsburgh: Intercultural Communication Network, Society For Intercultural Education Training and Research, 1972.

3

Psychological Aspects of Aging

Mary Kirchhofer and Marjorie Plumb

Throughout the centuries and in different cultures attitudes to aging have varied greatly. Some cultures have considered the physically weak and nonproductive elderly to be expendable, thus abandoning them to die unattended, while other cultures have cherished the old for their longevity and experience. Among early Native American societies, instances can be found both of cultures that revered the old and of cultures that systematically put the old to death. Older persons themselves have typically incorporated the expectations of their cultures. As recently as this century, in Japan, for example, old people went willingly (or even asked their unwilling sons to carry them) to special places in the hills, known as the Mountains of the Dead, where the old ones were left to die. In general, abandonment or ritual killing of the old has occurred in cultures that were hard-pressed for food and where the noncontributing individual was just another mouth to feed.[1] This treatment was not limited to the aged but was applied to the very sick and severely handicapped of these societies.

In contemporary America, people are living longer than ever before: birth rates have declined, and both the absolute and relative numbers of the elderly are steadily increasing. In 1982, Erikson was saying "A look back on this century's last few decades makes it clear that *old age* was 'discovered' only . . . when an ever-increasing number of old people were found to represent a mass of *elderlies* rather than an elite of *elders*."[2] The group growing most rapidly of all, those eighty-five years of age or older, inevitably includes the largest proportion of feeble, dependent persons and of physically and emotionally abused oldsters. It is this group that conforms most closely to negative stereotypes about age and aging; i.e., that old age must be a time of deteriorating health, disintegrating mind, and helpless dependency if not victimization. Yet, in actuality, even in this extreme age range there is a significant minority of persons managing quite well with little or no assistance.

Schaie and Willis (1986) have noted that it may be useful to distinguish among these "very-old" (late eighties and older), the "old-old" (late seventies/early eighties, most of whom still live in their own communities but with increasing problems), and the "young-old" (in their sixties and early seventies, retired but otherwise similar to persons of late middle age).[3] It is probably this latter "young-old" group, as well as fortunate individuals of the "old-old" and "very-old" groups, whose activities and financial circumstances are fostering what Gatz, Pearson, and Fuentes (1984)[4] refer to as a "countermyth" about old age. In contrast to the familiar negative stereotype, this new "countermyth" characterizes the old as shrewd, financially secure, comfortable with themselves, and generally enjoying life. Indeed, there is considerable evidence that sizable numbers of the elderly are both vital and vocal, quite able to challenge some of the assumptions of youth and to assert control over their own situations. The lifestyles of these individuals are often geared to physical fitness through sensible nutrition, exercise, and socialization. In recent years, many of them have become organized in associations with considerable lobbying power, which has made it possible for senior centers and congregate dining sites to be funded. Special rates and special programs for senior citizens also encourge travel, use of public parks, and attendance at cultural events. Entrepreneurs welcome seniors as customers and even in some cases as part-time paid employees. All in all, increased opportunities for stimulating activities and companionship, along with improved health practices, are helping more of the elderly to maintain themselves longer in good physical and mental condition, and to stay out of institutions.

CHRONOLOGICAL VERSUS DEVELOPMENTAL AGING

For any given age group, certain "norms" apply and certain facts are inescapable. Thus, for example, the current death rate of male American sixty-year-olds can be calculated with considerable accuracy, and is higher than the rate for ten year olds. Projections of the United States Office of the Actuary for the year 2000 estimate an average lifespan of slightly less than eighty-five years. According to Fries and Crapo, 95 percent of natural deaths will occur between the ages of seventy-seven and ninety-three, and only one person in 10,000 will reach the age of one hundred.[5] Even if death does not intervene, most people will experience a marked decline in their physical functioning somewhere between the ages of sixty-five and eighty. Nevertheless, useful as these statistical facts and figures are, they do not tell us *which* persons of the 10,000 will survive a century or more, and which persons in their eighties will be painting masterpieces. Precisely because of the variability among individuals who have lived the same number of years, it is important to try to distinguish *developmental age*—i.e., true mental and physical capacity to adapt and survive—from simple *chronological* age. As Kimmel observes, age-based entitlement programs inevitably reflect stereotypes and prejudices because "it is both too cumbersome and too costly for public policy to recognize the diversity,"[6] but diversity can and must be recognized in family and institutional decision making. In an ideal world, we would separate out the three factors of "norms" or averages, individual differences, and distortions of our understanding caused by ignorance or prejudice.

Interestingly, on almost all measures of physiological functioning, there is greater deviation from the average among the elderly, i.e., more variation, than there is among the twenty-to-thirty-year age group (Crapo and Fries, 1981). Most biological markers in fact correlate poorly with chronological age. The marker that correlates best is graying hair,[7] yet it is not unusual to see gray hair at age thirty (or at least it wasn't until hair coloring become acceptable and fashionable), and not uncommon for persons aged eighty or more to have very few gray hairs.

Physical changes are often offset by psychological attitudes. A person with wrinkled skin, slow or unsteady gait, and a stooped posture may be so alert mentally, have such charm and social poise that the chronological age is assumed to be younger than it is. Here it can be noted, too, that a number of studies of centenarians show them to have had exceptional mental as well as physical health, a sense of humor, and a capability for youthful enthusiasm. In the United States, "Visher studied two men of over 100 who were active, happy and seemingly in good health, although later their post mortems showed that several of their organs were diseased."[8]

Despite a recent explosion of gerontological research, there remain relatively few longitudinal studies of aging. Cross-sectional studies, especially when groups of widely disparate ages are compared, fail to take into account extraordinary changes in social environment during this century. Changes in working and housing conditions, nutrition, medical practices, sexual mores, retirement provisions, and so on, mean that each generation reaches its later years after a lifetime of experiences different from those of the generation before. As just one example of change, we know that large numbers of the generation who reached young adulthood in the 1960s chose to smoke marijuana rather than tobacco; the long-term health risks associated with tobacco are now well-understood while those associated with marijuana are still emerging.

According to Schaie (1988), a second flaw in many research designs is the failure to separate the effects of a disease from those of normal age changes. The danger of confounding age with generational differences and/or with disease is of course that false conclusions may be drawn from the research results and become the basis for public policy with its impact on the old.

FUNCTIONAL CHANGES

Birren and Zarit define psychological aging as "changes that occur in the ability of the organism to adapt its capacities; e.g., sensation, perception, memory, learning, intellectual abilities, drives and motivation, to alterations in the social and physical environment and within the organism itself."[9] What are some of the changes that affect function with increasing age? Very commonplace indeed are disturbances of sleep. Compared to younger groups, older persons have more difficulty falling asleep and staying asleep. According to Butler and Lewis, older persons experience less dreaming sleep. Deep sleep, the period of dreamless oblivion, lessens and may vanish in old age.[10] Old people who suffer from the aches and pains of degenerative disease, as well as anxiety and depression, may need more rather than less sleep. Insomnia is estimated to be a complaint of 90 percent of those aged sixty to eighty years.[11]

A second well-recognized problem is that there is some loss of memory as people age: the single most frequent complaint pertains to loss of memory for names. On the positive side, it has been shown that memory can improve with training, particularly in the use of retrieval clues. Langer and co-workers who studied nursing home patients averaging eighty years also found that interaction and rewards produced improvement in performance when several standard memory tests were given.[12]

Other factors that may influence the outcome of tests are the embarrassment and anxiety that older people may feel in the test situation, especially with younger people administering the tests. Indeed, emotions can interfere with memory at all ages. "*Recognition memory* (has been shown) not to deteriorate with age. Old people may have trouble with names and recalling facts out of context but they always recognize them when they see them again."[13] Environmental factors can also influence results. Data suggest that when the surroundings are drab, old people learn more slowly than their juniors, but when the tests are given in a bright and colorful room, results can be as good for the older as for the younger person.

Certain other types of cognitive performance have also been shown to respond favorably to preventive and remedial techniques. Even reaction time, which is known to slow with aging, is affected by the maintenance of physical fitness, and older persons benefit more from practice than their younger counterparts.[14] Schaie makes the further crucial point that age-related changes, as in reaction time, may indeed be well-documented and yet be quite unimportant in actual task performance. Due to experience or other compensatory mechanisms, the overall performance of the older person may be as good as that of the younger person, or so little slower that the deficit is of no practical significance.[15]

In response to the paucity of information on healthy aging as late as mid-century, a few investigators began studies from a wide range of research perspectives. The National Institute of Mental Health (NIMH) also undertook collaborative studies involving separate academic disciplines and medical specialties over a period of eleven years. The NIMH findings in general reinforced the hypothesis that much of what has been called aging is really disease. Arteriosclerosis rather than aging was found to be the probable cause of diminished blood flow to the brain. Healthy men with an average age of seventy-one presented cerebral function that compared favorably with a control group of men with an average age of twenty-one. For older persons, as for younger groups, current environmental satisfaction and support were found to be of critical import to psychological stability.[16]

The well-known behavioral psychologist B. F. Skinner has remarked from his own experience that "Old age is like fatigue, except that its effects cannot be corrected by relaxation or taking a vacation." Skinner proposes that what the aging individual needs is a "prosthetic environment," i.e., just as a person will use prosthetic devices such as eyeglasses or a hearing aid to make up for the loss of sensory acuity, so should the person try to arrange matters to compensate for his other failings. Skinner makes a number of suggestions to older people: for example, use memoranda to help out memory; do what you need to do as soon as it occurs to you and before you forget; become aware of the signs that mean that you are becoming tense or mentally weary (Skinner says that one such sign in himself is that he uses more profanity); when you have exhausted your old interests and/or can no longer keep up with them, find new things to take the place of the old—if necessary, soap operas instead of great literature.[17]

As Skinner sees it, so-called "lack of motivation" in old age is really a lack of positive reinforcements, i.e., rewards of pleasure and satisfaction for behavior. The old reinforcers are no longer easily available (since retirement, one rarely sees one's old colleagues), or do not work as well (food doesn't taste as good), or do not work at all (the brisk country hike produces aches and pains, so why hike in the future?). The solution is that one must find new reinforcers—new interests, new behaviors, new friends.

That self-confidence and self-esteem often come under sharp attack in old age seems undeniable. Devalued by younger people and cut off from many once-familiar gratifications, the old person can come to denigrate herself. Some evidence indicates that even their physicians tend to spend less time with aged patients than with younger ones.[18] The very clerks in the grocery store are apt to be more impatient with a slow old person than a slow young one. Sobel comments that "With advancing age, human relatedness becomes difficult . . . then the sense of worth, identity, and cohesiveness of the self begins to fall apart."[19] Meaningful, positive contacts with others are important too, for the perspectives and correctives they supply; they are windows to the world.

Community outreach efforts to support the sense of well-being, the reality testing, the physical health, and the self-sufficiency of older citizens have taken many forms, including some ingenious ones. For example, to overcome the shyness and suspiciousness of isolated old people living in inner-city hotel rooms, public health nurses in one community set up stations in the hotel lobbies. These stations not only provided free blood pressure check-ups but also began to function as informal meeting places where new friendships could be formed.[20] Programs that create or enhance opportunities for senior citizens to be useful may be especially crucial to morale: how many of the old have said, "I might as well be dead, I'm no good to anyone"? Sometimes the aged are quite ruthlessly burdened with work, typically with child-care duties that really are the responsibility of another generation, yet often the old are brushed aside and needlessly underutilized. Today there are women in their seventies caring for an aged parent while at the same time assisting in the care of grandchildren, but there are others who feel cast aside and they have no role at all.

Erikson, noted for his psychoanalytic theory of personality development based on psychosexual stages from infancy to old age, published *The Life Cycle Completed* when he was eighty. In his preface he says, "I . . . begin my account with the last one (stage), *old age*, to see how much sense a re-view of the *completed* life cycle can make of the whole course."[21] Such a review has been said by Butler "to provide new insight into experiences, wisdom that provides a better integrated, coherent picture of one who is in the late or last phase of his/her pilgrimage through life."[22]

Each of Erikson's eight stages builds upon earlier ones and each is characterized by a key issue that must be successfully resolved for optimal development. For example, in the infancy stage the issue is Basic Trust versus Mistrust, in adolescence it is Identity versus Identity Confusion, in maturity it is Creativity versus Stagnation, and in old age it is Integrity versus Despair. In old age, issues dealt with in the preceding seven stages are resolved. "It is the acceptance of one's one and only life cycle as something that had to be and that, by necessity, permitted no substitutions."[23] In *The Life Cycle Completed* (1980), Erikson tells how the theory of relativity helped him develop his psychosocial and historical theories, basing them always on psychoanalytic practice. He shows that the resolution of issues throughout the stages of his life has given him a sense of integrity, as he is able to conclude that "clinical work can supplement other ways of taking the pulse of changing history and in advancing an all-human awareness."[24]

Looking for "integrity" in old age, Kaufman took life stories from sixty elderly people, forty-eight of whom lived in their own homes and twelve of whom were in long-term care facilities. She learned that "In old age, people make new assessments of themselves as they create an integrated identity, account for the paths they have travelled, and formulate meaning for the rest of their lives."[25] She observed profound cultural issues in their lives: early poverty and the drive to overcome it by hard work, education as a means to financial reward and heightened self-esteem, assimilation for those who were immigrants. Nevertheless the meaning drawn from these experiences she found to be highly idiosyncratic. Today's middle-aged will undoubtedly have different experiences and values but will probably make the same effort to weave them into an integrated identity in old age.

DISENGAGEMENT VERSUS ACTIVITY

Is it more healthful for the elderly to remain active or to disengage from earlier involvements? While there is still some disagreement on these alternatives, the preponderance of studies indicate that psychological well-being is more likely to be the result of activity than of withdrawal. The elderly who perceive themselves as having control of future, personally important events show signs of vitality associated with activity; those who perceive events to be under external control or "fate" tend toward apathy and withdrawal.[26]

When Reker and Wong surveyed forty community and forty institutionalized elderly about their expectations for the future, it was clear that, for most, thinking revolved around family and how to spend leisure time. What was disquieting was the apparent lack of interest in personal change and development, possibly because of a belief in the myth that "you can't teach an old dog new tricks."[27] Lack of interest arising from this misconception should concern people interested in the well-being of the elderly since potential for growth is always present, regardless of age, provided only that there is the desire to grow.

To varying degrees, disengagement is forced upon many people by their physical limitations. Some have problems with driving after dark and must forego the meetings, concerts, plays, and volunteer work that had formed an important part of their earlier lives. Even if rides are offered, the individual's feeling of independence may be diminished. Impaired hearing often discourages attendance at church and lectures. Speakers are often unaware of the need to use a microphone, and the elderly do not always take advantage of the hearing aids available free in many churches and at theaters (for a small fee). Difficulty in understanding what others are saying may even inhibit the elderly in their everyday interactions with friends and neighbors. Obviously, in severe cases, limitations are more profound than these. An individual who is unable to communicate as a result of a stroke is likely to be cut off from almost everyone. A person who cannot walk even with a cane must depend on someone else to push a wheelchair, or rely on specialized equipment in order to get about at all. And, in both mild and severe cases, negative feelings about the self associated with the impairment may tend to exacerbate the actual physical difficulties.

Even for individuals in fairly good health, the economic environment is a major factor in maintaining an active lifestyle in old age. At no time in life is the possession of a truly adequate income more appreciated than in old age. To be able to leave a cold climate for a warm one, to travel freely and in comfort, to call for a cab as needed, to use medical services without undue worry about cost, to hire help when needed, make telephone calls as desired, and perhaps at the end to be cared for by nurses at home— all these enable the elderly person to feel in control and an active participant in life. A severely limited income often forces withdrawal and brings stresses that affect health.

SPECIFIC IMPAIRMENTS AFFECTING PSYCHOLOGICAL WELL-BEING

Hearing impairment, more common in the elderly than visual loss, according to Butler and Lewis, crucially affects mental health. About 75 percent of individuals in the seventy-to-seventy-nine age group have some degree of hearing loss, and it is more common among older men than older women.

Possibly, men are affected by higher decibels of noise in the workplace. However, profound hearing loss is more frequently found in women than in men. Both depression and paranoid ideation are common emotional consequences of hearing loss. Some antibiotics may be associated with damage to the inner ear, and diets high in saturated fats can also result in hearing loss. One study showed that hearing acuity improved with the substitution of polyunsaturated for saturated fats.[28] Presbycusis is the term used to describe hearing loss due to age-related changes in the inner ear, the auditory neural pathways, and the central auditory nervous system. It is likely that when the rock'n'roll generation reaches old age they will be suffering from sensorineural loss, since this damage is irreversible and occurs when there is exposure to noise at or above ninety decibels.

Visual impairment in older persons is usually caused by presbyopia, the result of diminished elasticity of the crystalline lens. When this is corrected by glasses, 80 percent of older people have reasonably good sight until age ninety or beyond. Diminished ability to adapt to darkness is common and requires proper lighting, especially night lights. White paint or strips of white materials outlining steps can give reassurance and avert many a fall. Common causes of blindness in people over sixty-five are macular degeneration*, cataracts, glaucoma, and diabetic retinopathy. Butler feels it is important for nonmedical mental health teams to learn the common physical symptoms of eye problems to avoid putting a psychiatric label on a physical process, and to increase empathy and understanding. For example, colored halos around lights are a common symptom of glaucoma and should not be interpreted as an illusion.[29] When severe hearing impairment is combined with loss of sight, communication becomes a critical problem. Touch then becomes an essential tool for breaking through the social isolation that occurs.

Overmedication. Although older people make up 11 percent of the population, they consume 25 percent of all medications prescribed in the United States as well as massive amounts of over-the-counter medications.[30] Guttman (1977) listed the four categories of drugs most frequently prescribed for the elderly as tranquilizers, diuretics, cardiovascular drugs, and sedatives/hypnotics. Among people living in the community, he found that the drugs were mostly taken as prescribed, but roughly half of those in the study combined their prescriptions with over-the-counter drugs and/ or alcohol.[31] Among those taking only prescribed drugs there was still considerable multiple drug use, leading to damaging overmedication. Not

---

*Refers to the breakdown of the macula lutea, a spot in the eye near the retina that is the center of visual keenness.—Eds.

even the institutionalized are immune to the risk of side effects from overmedication. One study of medication used in a proprietary nursing home showed a total of 536 prescriptions for 98 patients; one patient received a total of 16 different drugs. The average number of PRN (as needed) prescriptions was 3.2 per patient. The overmedication of the old is all the more extraordinary in view of the fact that drug studies have very rarely used subjects in their seventies and eighties.

Overmedication in the United States today affects all age groups and is caused by the tendency of the mass media, physicians, families of patients, and the pharmaceutical industry to see pills as the cure for most human ailments. However, for the elderly the danger of damage is far higher as a result of changes in absorption, distribution, metabolism, and excretion that accompany aging. Also the lack of appropriate psychological intervention, which results from ignorance and misunderstanding on the side of both the provider and the recipient, leads to unnecessary pharmacological intervention.

This is not to imply that all medication is overmedication or that all so-called "psychological" interventions are effective. Studies suggest that in reality orientation therapy the significant factor was not any specific procedure or intervention the therapist brought to bear but rather the overall quality of the patient-therapist relationship. Familiar social activities such as wine drinking and dancing have been found to enhance feelings of well-being and to facilitate normal socialization patterns. In cases of far advanced dementia, Feil finds "validation" to be helpful. Rather than insisting on present reality, she follows the patient's need to talk, perhaps of mother and childhood. This, according to Feil, has a tranquilizing and normalizing effect on even highly disturbed patients.[32]

RELATIONSHIPS WITH HEALTH PROFESSIONALS

Jahningen, Head of the Section of Geriatric Medicine of the Cleveland Clinic Foundation (1987), has provided an interesting discussion of patient relationships with a variety of health-care providers.[33] He compares the "provider-client" relationship of the elderly with social workers, noninstitutional nurses, occupational therapists, etc., with the "patient-doctor" and "patient-nurse" relationship in hospitals. A client-provider type of relationship implies substantial freedom of choice by the client, with the professional providing advice or service. The patient-doctor relationship, on the other hand, usually involves less autonomy for the "patient." The physician assigns the individual a "sick" role, thus acknowledging that the person is ill through no fault of his own, and permitting both the patient and his relatives and friends to accept dependency on the physician. Jahningen quite rightly states that "society accords physicians authority, as it does policemen, teachers, priests, and presidents," but it is also true that in many circumstances social workers and others may be perceived as having considerable power and knowledge. In practice the client may also defer to their authority.

The type of relationship the individual has with any "health care provider" will obviously be the outcome of a variety of factors, including the kind and degree of the individual's need, the personalities of all concerned, previous experiences of the individual with health caregivers, and so on. For example, some individuals reject dependence while others welcome it.

The wellness movement of the 1970s and 1980s, which stresses responsibility for one's own health, has led to an increase in questioning the physician's authority in both health and disease. Because nutrition, exercise, and prevention generally have not been emphasized in medical training until recently, the physician has not necessarily been a good and readily available source of information on preventing ill health. Through the press and television, however, a great deal of information about the body and its healthy functioning and about various types of illness and treatment is being made available to broad segments of the population. More old persons as well as younger ones are taking greater responsibility for their own states of health and for making treatment decisions.

MENTAL HEALTH CONSULTATION IN PHYSICAL ILLNESS

Dr. Lebowitz of the National Institute of Mental Health (1987) states that "A basic tenet of geriatric care is, or at least should be, that all potentially disabling conditions have behavioral, emotional, and therefore, mental health components."[34] A striking phrase here is "at least should be." Almost everyone would agree with Dr. Lebowitz in theory. In practice the emotional and mental-health aspects of physical illness and disability are likely to be disregarded unless the patient is either profoundly depressed or seriously disruptive because of panic or bizarre behavior. Lebowitz argues that mental-health interventions should be seen as essential components of hospital care for all older persons, and suggests that one result in many cases would be reduced length of hospital stay. Indeed, if the importance of consultation and liaison with mental-health disciplines is genuinely accorded an integral part in the care of seniors with significant medical illness, good mental health may accompany the medical prolongation of life in this century.

FEAR OF DEATH AND DYING

For many older people, and certainly those in the old-old age group, death itself is not nearly so much feared as prolongation of dying. Indeed, death is often welcomed as a release from suffering or sometimes simply from the sense of being a burden to loved ones. While medical knowledge and technology (along with costs) have increased astronomically in the last fifty years, the medical profession has not yet fully integrated its power to prolong life with its mission to relieve suffering. At times the two seem to be at odds. Fortunately the hospice movement, which originated in England for the care of the terminally ill cancer patient, is now influencing the medical profession's attitude to dying from all causes. The essential goal of hospice is to enable the terminally ill patient to live out his days as fully as possible. This is accomplished by providing pain relief without regard to addiction or shortening of life and by assisting the family in keeping the patient at home until the end, when possible. When this is not possible, Hospice provides free-standing institutions with few regulations, where visitors, children, even pets, can come at any time of the day or night.

Contrary to the hospice philosophy that accepts death as a natural passage through the journey of life, many physicians and other medical personnel equate death with failure. They are trained to think that life must be sustained through all possible measures even if these require the loss of human dignity and freedom of choice. Family and friends often concur or even insist on such measures, perhaps through feelings of guilt or perhaps the conviction that living at any price is better than surrender to death. The threat of malpractice, unfortunately, can also influence the physician's behavior. Thus a patient in a nursing home may be suffering mentally and physically and longing to die, yet every time death approaches, the nursing home sends him or her off to the hospital for intensive care, and longed-for death is once more postponed.

Probably the greatest fear the elderly have is of loss of control resulting from strokes with aphasia or senile dementia. Especially is this so for those in good mental health who are in long-term care institutions where the preponderance of patients have been admitted because of Alzheimer's or related dementias. It is reassuring for the mentally healthy but otherwise incapacitated individual to know that there are ways in which she can arrange for her wishes to be carried out even in the event of incompetence. Two instruments that she can use are a durable power of attorney and a living will, both of which remain in effect even if she becomes incapacitated, and are available in all of the states and in the District of Columbia. (In contradistinction, a general power of attorney becomes effective only when an individual is *declared* incompetent.) Forms for a living will, available from the Euthanasia Education Council,* specify "that medication be mercifully administered to me to alleviate suffering even though this may hasten the moment of death" and are intended specifically for the attending physician but can also be shared with any family or friend who should know the person's wishes. A living will based on a durable power of attorney "can grant very broad powers and, in effect, can be used to transfer all the legal capacity of the principal to another person, the attorney-in-fact, who will act in the principal's place."[35] It can also limit those powers so that the attorney-in-fact has only the powers granted him in the living will.

MENTAL/EMOTIONAL DISORDERS

In addition to experiencing the effects of normal aging processes, many of the aged suffer from specific mental/emotional disorders of varying severity. In old age, such disorders often result from physical damage to the nervous system or from patho-physiological conditions, or both. An older individual may, however, also have psychological disturbance when there is little or no evidence of damage in the brain, or a disturbance may antedate such evidence. Perhaps the individual has a long history of psychiatric problems, either mild or very serious. Or the patient may have functioned well throughout most of her life and become disturbed only in response to exceptional stresses in old age.

In mental disorders, the brain tissue itself may be healthy or not, and may be affected temporarily or permanently. In the case of some disorders, the brain is apparently normal and the disorders seem to be the outcome of psychological or social factors. In the case of other disorders, it is suspected but cannot yet be demonstrated that the brain chemistry is awry. Still other disorders are linked quite clearly to dysfunction of the brain. These latter are the "organic mental disorders," some of which are common in the elderly.

Among the sixty-five and older group, dementia is the most frequently seen of the various brain dysfunctions. In dementia, the crucial feature is a loss of intellectual abilities severe enough to interfere with social or occupational functioning. Depending on how far the dementia has progressed, there will be impairment not only of memory but also of concentration, problem solving, judgment, capacity to learn, orientation, language, and motor skills. Emotional control may deteriorate, personality may change, and behavior becomes mildly to grossly inappropriate.

---

*250 W. 57th Street, New York, NY 10019

When the picture of dementia is recognized in an elderly person, it is tempting to jump to the conclusion that the mental failings are irreversible, but this is not the only possibility. There may, for example, have been a severe, acute medical problem superimposed on a very mild chronic state. If acute conditions are ignored, the person may needlessly deteriorate into severe dementia, and a treatable underlying illness may be missed with disastrous results.

Although reversible causes of dementia must always be ruled out, it is true that most dementias in the elderly are associated either with Alzheimer's disease or with brain damage from multiple occlusion of small cerebral arteries.[36] It is not always possible to recognize the onset of irreversible dementias. Both family and the individuals themselves are anxious to attribute symptoms to "normal" aging processes. It is often only in hindsight that aberrant behavior, occurring months or even over a year earlier, is recognized as having been the onset of either Alzheimer's disease or the first episode in multi-infarct dementia (dementia as a result of blood shortage to the brain).

Alzheimer's disease has an insidious onset and typically a rather slow but relentlessly deteriorating course. At the very beginning, the individual may merely seem to have minor difficulty recalling names or where things were put, but as the memory deficit worsens, it becomes clear that more than benign age-related forgetfulness is involved. According to Reisberg and Ferris, a "confusional phase" may be ushered in by an incident in which the person becomes lost while traveling and cannot sort out what needs to be done or in which she forgets important business or social matters.[37] When she recognizes that she is having problems, the person may at first be overtly quite upset. At a later point, as recent memory suffers more and more and other cognitive abilities fade, the person may refuse to admit that anything is wrong. She may at times "confabulate" or invent answers to memory questions, either without apparent awareness that she is inventing, or consciously, to cover embarrassment. Gradually, behavior of all kinds is likely to become more idiosyncratic and less subject to social constraints: the woman who was once meticulous in her grooming becomes slatternly and wears the same odd garments day after day; the man who was a model of propriety becomes the "dirty old man" who exhibits himself on a street corner.

When the day comes on which the individual can no longer manage to function independently even in a marginal way, she is said to have reached the "dementia" stage.[38] By this time the person is no longer in adequate contact with reality. She may retain only childhood memories and come to behave as if she were in fact living in the past. Finally, the individual may forget even her own name, how to feed herself, how to walk. We say, then, that the person we used to know is no longer there. Although there is as yet no treatment for Alzheimer's disease, associated bizarre behavioral disturbances—delusions, hallucinations, agitation, and violence—can be controlled by antipsychotic drugs. Since it is often these behaviors that necessitate institutionalization, drug treatment may enable the family to keep the individual at home. Dr. Reisberg, who headed a New York University team that studied fifty-seven Alzheimer's patients, cautions that these patients respond to much lower drug dosages than younger patients. He emphasizes that physicians today can greatly ease the suffering caused by the disease by treating the treatable symptoms.[39]

Although some disagreement exists among experts, the typical estimate is that 4 to 6 percent of persons sixty-five and older have Alzheimer's disease, while 50 to 60 percent of senile dementias are thought to be of the Alzheimer's type.[40] Based on several survey studies, Gatz and Pearson conclude that most people believe Alzheimer's disease is more prevalent than is actually the case.[41] They suggest that the very emphasis on Alzheimer's in the media "may have an unintended consequence . . . older adults may become hyperaware of their own lapses and needlessly fear that they are developing the disease." Not only older adults themselves but also those who are their potential caretakers dread what may happen.

Indeed, during the long slow decline of Alzheimer's, the family is typically highly stressed and in great need of support. This need is being met to some extent by the organization known as the Alzheimer's Disease and Related Disorders Association (ADRDA) of which there are many small groups around the country.* Psychosocial help is also available. Adult day-care centers often make it possible for the family to keep the individual suffering from Alzheimer's living at home, thus postponing institutionalization until near the end. Some nursing homes also offer "respite care"; they admit the patient for a week or two so that the family can take a vacation. Many caregiver classes are also now available that teach ways of coping.

Multi-infarct dementia is also irreversible and has only fairly recently been differentiated from Alzheimer's type dementia. In fact the two sometimes occur together. The progress of this disease is more erratic and less predictable than the slow, steady deterioration of Alzheimer's type. A great deal of research is being done on these diseases and diagnosis is being facilitated to some extent by the development of new technology, such as positron emission tomography (PET) and nuclear magnetic resonance (NMR). However, these new techniques are extremely expensive.

---

*360 N. Michigan Avenue, Room 601, Chicago, IL, 60601

Like dementia, delirium occurs frequently in the elderly, is likely to involve extensive cognitive impairment, and must always be taken seriously. Delirious persons as well as the demented display disturbances of memory, reasoning, perception, speech, psychomotor activity, and emotional control. Delirium, however, differs from dementia in several ways.

First, in delirium disordered attention and wakefulness are major symptoms.[42] Second, delirium is transient, lasting usually about a week and rarely more than a month, while dementia due to Alzheimer's disease and/or multiple infarcts is chronic. Dementia's onset is insidious but delirium's onset is rapid. Sometimes delirium's onset is the first warning sign of an underlying physical illness, while in other instances it seems to be a response to an external stressor such as bereavement. The outcome of advanced degenerative dementia is death. Delirium, if neglected and severe, may also be fatal, but prompt and proper treatment often clears up the condition. Third, the symptoms of dementia are likely to be quite stable over the short-run but those of delirium tend to fluctuate sharply. It is extremely important to differentiate between reversible and irreversible dementia. For instance, reversible disorders may be the result of malnutrition, overmedication, tumor, hydrocephalus, or depression.[43,44]

Depression may be mistaken for an organic brain syndrome since certain symptoms of depression, especially if severe, create a picture that is superficially quite similar.[45] There may in fact be a high incidence of elderly depressed persons misdiagnosed as demented. In one recent study, 28 percent of patients who were referred to a clinic as "demented" were found instead to be suffering from depression.[46]

One reason for diagnostic confusion is simply that the symptoms of depression are so varied and may appear in so many combinations. Prominent somatic symptoms are loss of appetite with marked weight loss not otherwise explained; disruption in sleep patterns, especially early morning awakening; easier fatigability; constipation; changes in the person's customary pace of thinking, speaking, and acting, typically in the direction of slowing down but sometimes in the direction of an agitated speeding up. Concurrent with such symptoms there may be social withdrawal, irritability, boredom, brooding, indecisiveness, or apathy about things that previously mattered. There may be somewhat paranoid or hypochondriacal preoccupation with body functions. There are sometimes frequent crying spells without clear cause, and feelings of dejection, worthlessness, guilt, and despair perhaps to the point of suicidal thoughts. Suicidal thoughts and feelings are not infrequent, and indeed the rate of completed suicide for men over sixty-five is four times higher than for the general population, while for women over sixty-five it is twice as high.[47] "Alarming as these statistics are, they probably represent a drastic underreporting. The elderly can easily disguise suicide by taking overdoses of drugs, failing to continue with life-sustaining medication, or starving themselves."[48]

For a variety of reasons, older persons may be less willing than younger persons to admit negative feelings about themselves and their life circumstances. Thus, when an older person looks despondent or suddenly behaves in uncharacteristic ways or constantly complains of vague health problems despite medical reassurances, the possibility of depression and even suicidal intentions should always be investigated. Increased consumption of alcohol can be a clue that the person is distressed. It should also be kept in mind that depression is sometimes an early symptom of serious physical illness, e.g., cancer of the pancreas, and often accompanies it.[49]

One explanation for the relatively high incidence of depression among the old is that depression is in fact a normal reaction to loss. The older person may be grieving for what she once was as well as what she once had. Sometime in the decade between the ages of sixty and seventy, most people voluntarily or involuntarily give up their work-related roles and the structure and prestige those roles provided. More and more as the years pass, friends and relatives depart. Loss of a spouse with whom the person has shared most of a lifetime is especially traumatic, and some old people outlive the middle-aged children on whom they were depending. Individuals may also grieve in anticipation of further losses that they cannot help but foresee.

Anxiety. Similarly, tension and fear are normal reactions to situations perceived as dangerous. As the capacities for self-maintenance and sources of self-esteem erode, it is understandable that fear and distrust should develop. It is only when depression, fear, and suspicion are markedly disproportionate to reality, or when these feelings themselves seriously interfere with coping capacity, that they should be considered symptoms of mental illness.

Both ordinary fearfulness and clinical states of anxiety can sometimes be seen in elderly persons. The symptoms of anxiety can be of any degree of intensity and can fluctuate over time for the same individual. Symptoms range from very mild to so powerful that the afflicted person is overwhelmed by terror and feelings of imminent death or insanity. At the panic end of the spectrum, there may be marked physical symptoms such as muscular tension, nausea, diarrhea, lump in the throat, light-headedness, trembling, dry mouth, or rapid pulse.[50]

If of a mild degree, anxiety can arouse and prod people to do things that need to be done. Too much anxiety, though, is counterproductive. Interfering as it does with memory, concentration, judgment, and decision making, anxiety can exacerbate the cognitive deficits of old people and heighten their vulnerability. Anxiety over their financial resources has made some old people fall victim to swindlers and others to become fanatical hoarders of junk. Anxiety that nursing homes will run out of space has made still others enter such facilities quite prematurely.[51] Severe panic attacks are so disruptive and aversive that people, whether young or old, who have had them become very fearful about the possibility of having more, and will resort to control measures such as staying shut up inside their houses for months at a time.

TREATMENT

Symptoms of anxiety and/or depression, whether recognized as such or not, are one of the most common reasons for people to visit primary care physicians. The elderly especially are far more likely to consult a family doctor or internist than a psychiatrist, although it has been noted that this is changing in the population that will form the aged in the next century. As suggested earlier, the increased incidence of medical problems plus mental/emotional distress in old people means that they consume several times as much medical care as the younger adult population, and that a disproportionately high percentage of psychotropic drug prescriptions (tranquilizers, antidepressants, etc.) are written for the over-sixty-five age group. Old people tend to comply poorly with physicians' instructions and will sometimes mix and match their medications quite promiscuously and sometimes dangerously, either out of confusion or naivete. Physicians should investigate what, if any, over-the-counter drugs are being used, and should take time to give careful and explicit instructions on how to take both prescribed and over-the-counter drugs. Clearly written instructions are best, since verbal instructions may not be remembered correctly.

It was noted above that the elderly are far more likely to consult a family doctor than a psychiatrist for help with emotional distress. Most people in fact take their personal troubles to others who are not mental health professionals. Quite apart from natural reticence and worries about being considered "crazy" for consulting mental health professionals, older persons may fail to seek treatment for reasons such as lack of insurance coverage and/or confusing regulations and paperwork requirements for reimbursement. Congressman Roybal comments that "Medicare psychiatric benefits . . . are outmoded and markedly inferior to benefits for physical illness," and points out that outpatient psychiatric benefits and in-nursing home mental health services are both "virtually nonexistent."[52] Furthermore, only a very small percentage of persons served either by community mental health centers or by private therapists are senior citizens. The negative (and inaccurate) view of certain mental health providers that the old are less likely to benefit from psychiatric treatment than the young erects still another barrier. The upshot is that older portions of the population do not begin to receive adequate mental health services.

Fortunately, there are some indications that today's adults in the twenty to forty-nine year range are more receptive than their elders to seeking help for emotional problems and may carry that attitude over to their own later years. In addition, pressure is growing on insurance companies and government agencies to offer more reasonable support for mental health services.

When older persons are being cared for in situations such as sheltered housing, nursing homes, or hospitals, much of the emotional help and support they receive will be provided by paraprofessional and nonprofessional staff, by the nurse's aide or the maintenance man or the volunteer who delivers the flowers. At times, help of value—some encouraging word or comforting gesture—won't be labeled as such because it will be given so spontaneously and unself-consciously. At other times, one or another staff person will take on unmistakable special significance for an older individual. This staff member may receive the confessions of overt anxiety or anger, which the individual is too proud to make, or does not dare to make, to family or physician.

A number of therapists have pointed out that distressed older persons will consciously or unconsciously behave so as to try to maximize caring and support from others. They may exaggerate their woes as a claim on sympathy or seek to be ingratiating or try to impress others with their importance or threaten retribution if support is not forthcoming. In the effort to preserve their dignity, they may, on the other hand, deny even blatant disabilities or blame them on others, or they may increasingly avoid even many activities or responsibilities they could still manage well. Unfortunately, it must be admitted that the staff in many institutions encourage dependence, finding it easier and quicker to do *for* the patient, rather than taking the time to let them try to do what they can do for themselves.

GUIDELINES

It will come as no surprise that there is no single best way to work with psychologically troubled older persons, no easy formula to plug in. Some useful guidelines, though, are these:

1. Assess the person's *unique* situation with care. Is this a fairly intact older person who can function independently with just a little practical help? Someone who is physically disabled but very alert?

Someone so depressed and agitated that she cannot think straight? Someone severely and irreversibly demented? Get as much history as possible about what the person was like in the past and what has been happening recently. Make use of the observations of as many different people as possible. Never assume that an assessment is forever, but make sure it is updated from time to time. Keep a sharp eye out for changes.

2. Try to understand what the person's particular concerns and coping mechanisms are. Remember that outraged complaints about minor ailments or injustices may be disguised expressions of underlying fears of sickness, abandonment, or death. Observe how the person tries to preserve her self-esteem and help with that when you reasonably can. Don't try to undo the person's denial of things that may be too painful to face.

3. Recognize that the person's mental functioning and emotional control may be quite variable, depending on such factors as fatigue and mood and physical ease. Be flexible in how you interact with her. Mothering the person may be appropriate at one time, but uncalled for at another time.

4. Help the person to retain as much independence and sense of control as possible. People develop many little strategies to help them cope—special places where they put things and small rituals they follow to enhance feelings of security—and these schemes should rarely be disturbed. Even in—or perhaps particularly in—a nursing home or hospital setting, the person's sense of control can often be heightened by quite simple things, e.g., by asking the person if it is all right to move her from the bed to the wheelchair before in fact moving her, by letting the person set her own pace in what she does, by preparing her for what may be about to happen next, etc. Don't just swoop down, because this may alarm or disturb her. Give explanations and time for adjustment.

   Support the person's sense of self-worth. Provide whatever opportunities possible for the person to be useful by helping others or perhaps simply by contributing to her own care. Try to arrange situations where she can make a choice or a decision. See to it that the person has at least a little privacy. Take the person seriously, e.g., don't make promises that can't be kept. Be affectionate if sincere, but avoid the condescending pat on the back.

   A seemingly minor but in fact important matter is that of how you address the individual. Explore the most supportive way to address the person, i.e., what name to use. Use of the individual's first name without specified permission is sometimes considered an invasion of privacy, and many people resent and find demeaning the use of terms like "dear" or "honey" unless a close relationship has in fact developed. On the other hand, some people are uncomfortable when addressed formally as "Mr." or "Mrs." or "Miss."

Help the person present as physically attractive a picture as possible. In short, think of the sorts of things that increase feelings of self-esteem and remember how much everyone depends on the respect she receives.

5. Try to be aware of your own attitudes and anxieties and those of others who are involved with the person. There is no question but that handicapped and seriously ill and/or aged people elicit fears in others about their own vulnerability and weakness and that these fears in turn often lead to avoidance behavior. There is also no question but that most people tend to be judgmental. If a person's problems are thought to be no fault of her own, then care providers are likely to be generous with their help than when they decide that someone brought the troubles on herself. One final example of the effect of attitudes: because of rigid or naive ideas about the sexual feelings of older people, barriers to perfectly natural exchanges of affection are set up. While it is not always possible to remake anxieties and attitudes, keeping them in mind is instructive. Sometimes a problem can be with the service provider and not with the older person at all.

6. Although it can help to simplify the environment and maintain orderly routines that the older person can count on, routines should not be inflexible. People should know what to expect, but one expectation should be that unusual circumstances will be recognized and a response forthcoming. The depriving iron hand of an institution or program isn't really necessary. Seemingly minor concessions, flexibilities, and comforts can mean a lot.

7. With the best motives at all times, it is not possible to remake the world. Decide what one person can reasonably accomplish and mobilize others to assist whenever possible.

Much work with the aged, as with the ill and disabled of all ages, involves sadness. Understand that sometimes the most important thing is to listen or simply be around, and this can be more helpful than one might think. People, when they complain, don't always expect or even want to have all their problems solved. When reasonable solutions are offered they may say "Yes but. . . ." What is wanted/expected/needed is attention, simple presence, and the acknowledgment that they matter. If very seriously impaired, old people may not comprehend what is said or recognize who said it, but gentleness is always recognized.

REFERENCES

1. deBeauvoir, Simone. *The Coming of Age* (trans.) New York: G. P. Putnam's Sons, 1972, pp. 38-87.

2. Erikson, Erik H. *The Life Cycle Completed.* New York: W. W. Norton & Co., 1982, p. 9.

3. Schaie, K. Warner. "Ageism in Psychological Research." *American Psychologist* (March 1988): 180.

4. Ibid., p. 186.

5. Fries, James F., and Crapo, Lawrence M. *Vitality and Aging.* San Francisco, Calif.: W. H. Freeman & Co., 1981, p. 77.

6. Kimmel, Douglas C. *American Psychologist,* (March 1988): 175.

7. Fries and Crapo, loc. cit. p. 108.

8. deBeauvoir, op. cit. p. 545.

9. Birren, James E., and Zarit, Judy M. "Concepts of Health, Behavior, and Aging," in Birren, J. E., and Livingston, J. (eds.) *Cognition, Stress, and Aging.* Englewood Cliffs, N.J.: Prentice-Hall 1985, p. 9.

10. Butler, Robert N., and Lewis, Myrna L. *Aging and Mental Health.* (3d ed.) St. Louis, Mo.: The C. V. Mosby Co., 1982, p. 378.

11. Reynold, C. F., Kupfer, D. J., and Sewitch, D. "Diagnosis and Management of Sleep Disorders in the Elderly." *Hospital and Community Psychiatry* 35 (1984): 779-781.

12. Fries and Crapo, op. cit., p. 118.

13. Oberleder, M. *Avoiding the Aging Trap.* Washington, D.C.: Acropolis Books Ltd., 1982, p. 22.

14. Fries and Crapo, op. cit., p. 116.

15. Schaie, op. cit., p. 181.

16. Butler, R. N., and Lewis, M. *Aging and Mental Health.* Rev., 1983, p. 11.

17. Skinner B. F. "Intellectual Self Management in Old Age." *American Psychologist* (1983): 239-244.

18. Vandenbos, G. R., and Buchanan, J. "Aging, Research on Aging, and National Policy: A Conversation with Robert Butler." *American Psychologist* (1983): 300-307.

19. Sobel, E. F. "Anxiety and Stress in Later Life." In Kitash, I. L., Schlesinger L. B. and Associates (eds.). *Handbook on Stress and Anxiety.* San Francisco, Calif.: Jossey-Bass Inc., 1980, pp. 317-328.

20. Pilisuk, M., and Minkler, M. "Supportive Networks: Life Ties for the Elderly." *Journal of Social Issues* 36 (1980): 95-116.

21. Erikson, E. H. 1982, loc. cit., p. 9.

22. Butler, R. N., Introduction in Quigley, P. *Those Were the Days.* Buffalo, N.Y.: Potentials Development, Inc., 1981.

23. Erikson E. H. *Childhood and Society.* New York: W. W. Norton, 1963.

24. ———, *The Life Cycle Completed,* p. 103.

25. Kaufman, S. R. *The Ageless Self.* New York: New American Library/Penguin, 1987, p. 186.

26. Shupe, D. R. "Perceived Control, Helplessness, and Choice." In Birren, J. E., and Livingston J. (eds.), op. cit., p. 161.

27. Reker, G. T., and Wong, T. P. "Personal Optimism: Physical and Mental Health." In Birren, J. E., and Livingston J. (eds.), loc. cit., p. 161.

28. Verrillo, R. T., and Verrillo V. "Sensory and Perceptual Performance." In Charress, N. (ed.). *Aging & Human Performance.* New York: J. Wiley & Sons, 1955, p. 9.

29. Butler, R. N., and Lewis M. L., op. cit., p. 111.

30. Ibid., op. cit., p. 292.

31. Levy, S. M., Derogatis, L. R., Gallagher, D., and Gatz, M. "Intervention with Older Adults and the Evaluation of Outcome." In Poon, L. W. (ed.), *Aging in the 1980s,* loc. cit., p. 45.

32. Feil, N. (1982).

33. Jahnigen, D. "The Changing Doctor-Patient Relationship." *Journal of the American Society on Aging* 12, no. 1, (1987): 54.

34. Lebowitz, B. D. (NIMH). "Mental Health Policy and Aging," p. 53.

35. Alexander, G. J. "Keeping Control with the Versatile Living Will." *Perspective on Aging,* NCOA, (July/August 1987): 20.

36. Wells, C. "Chronic Brain Disease: An Update on Alcoholism, Parkinson's Disease, and Dementia." *Hospital and Community Psychiatry* 33 (1982): 111-126.

37. Reisberg, B., and Ferris, S. H. "Diagnosis and Assessment of the Older Patient." *Hospital and Community Psychiatry* 33 (1982): 104-110.

38. Ibid.

39. *O. T. Week,* AOTA National Weekly, 1988, (March 10, 1988): 2.

40. Terry and Katzman (1983) cited in *American Psychologist* (March 1988): 186.

41. *American Psychologist,* op. cit., p. 184.

42. Lipowski, Z. T. "Transient Cognitive Disorders (Delirium, Acute Confusional States) in the Elderly." *American Journal of Psychiatry* 140 (1983): 1426-1436.

43. Maletta, G. J., Pirozzolo, F. J., Thompson, G., and Mortimer, J. A. "Organic Mental Disorders in a Geriatric Outpatient Population." *American Journal of Psychiatry* 139 (1982): 521-158.

44. Brown, D. S. *Handle with Care—A Question of Alzheimer's.* Buffalo, N.Y.: Prometheus Books in cooperation with Potentials Development, 1984, p. 24.

45. Thompson, T. L., Morgan, M. G., and Nies, A. S. "Psychotropic Drug Use in the Elderly." *The New England Journal of Medicine* 308 (1983): 134, 138, 194-199.

46. Maletta, G. J., et al., op. cit.

47. Resnik, H. L. P., and Cantor, J. M. "Suicide and Aging." *Journal of American Geriatrics Society* 18 (1970): 152-158.

48. Holland, J. "Psychological Aspects of Cancer Medicine." In Holland, J. F., and Frei, E. (eds.), *Cancer Medicine.* Philadelphia: Lea & Febiger, 1982.

49. Ibid.

50. *Diagnostic and Statistical Manual of Mental Disorders* (3d ed.). The American Psychiatric Association, 1980.

51. Ibid.

52. Roybal, E. R. "Agenda for the 100th Congress." *Journal of the American Society on Aging* 12, no. 1 (1987): 72.

FOR DISCUSSION TOPICS

1. List three differences between depression and dementia.

2. List three things that characterize older people according to the new counter-myth of old age.

3. List three things that characterize older people according to the myth of old age.

4. What two pursuits of the current younger generation are most likely to lead to disabilities in old age? What would these disabilities be?

4

Physical Aspects of Aging

David H. Dube

INTRODUCTION

Aging in the United States is accompanied by profound social and physiologic changes. Without a thorough understanding of such changes, physicians who care for elderly patients may be less effective than when armed with such knowledge. Not only can normal physiological changes with age be confused with disease processes, but disease manifestations can also be masked by a variety of aging processes. Additionally, understanding the complex interactions between patients, their environments, and caregivers must be incorporated into the formulation of proper medical and social treatment plans.

GENERAL CONSIDERATIONS

Social programs, insurance, and economic issues impact upon physicians' abilities to care for their patients. Such programs may change from state to state, or even between cities or counties within a given state. Specialized diets, for example, may be required for adequate treatment of a medical condition; if a patient is unable to acquire such a diet, the medical problem may be aggravated. If a specialized meal service is available in the community and the physician is unaware of such a resource, the doctor will not be effective in the delivery of care to his elderly patient who has special dietary requirements.

Not only must the geriatrician understand complex patient-related issues, so too, he or she must be linked to the network of services available for patients within their immediate and extended environments. Such linkages come from senior centers, departments of social service, state and local governmental programs for the aged (generally found in the phone book), and, most importantly, such linkages are established through daily attempts to listen and respond to the individual needs of the patients. The geriatrician soon learns which consulting physicians have handicapped access to their offices. More importantly, that geriatrician learns to ask before referring the patient if the patient will be physically able to enter the office to which they might be referred.

For the frail elderly, the physician must develop a capacity to learn about and respond to the support systems available to each patient. Despite a commonly held notion that most frail elderly are in long-term care facilities, most studies show that frail patients are often cared for by an extended family support network, and nursing home placement is only precipitated after "caretaker burnout." Had the physician been more responsive to the caretaker needs, such "burnout" might have been prevented by provision of timely support services. Such support services might include home aides or even introduction of a "respite" program. Respite programs allow fatigued caretakers to take much-needed breaks from the heavy demand of twenty-four-hour caregiving by temporarily placing the patient in a chronic care respite setting.

Some diseases associated with aging can be especially taxing on care providers. One such illness is dementia. These patients lose all kinds of abilities and eventually become bedridden, total-care patients. The disease progression generally takes years. It is easy to understand how much work toileting, dressing, feeding, grooming, positioning in bed, and total hygiene might be in the later stages of dementia. But, imagine how much more difficult patients might be to handle when they are in the early stages of dementia, unable to ever be safely left alone, with reversed day and night sleep cycles, constant repetitions of the same questions, and extreme emotional volatility. Such patients might only demonstrate agitation as a manifestation of a severe medical problem. Often the only person aware of such changes in the health status of demented patients is the caregiver. Those caregivers must then provide the physician with the nonspecific symptoms of an illness. Imagine how difficult it becomes for the physician when direct questioning of the patient is not possible and the only symptom the caregiver might complain of is that the patient isn't "acting right" or perhaps she just doesn't "look good."

As stated elsewhere in this volume, women outlive men in our society. It is a sad fact that the fastest-growing segment of poor in our society is the newly widowed woman who has faithfully nursed a husband through the last stages of a terminal illness and is subsequently impoverished by the large expenses of such care. Well over 50 percent of the entire Medicare budget is spent on the last months of life. Without any knowledge of such social realities, physicians can often find themselves, with all good intentions, being the unwitting agents of impoverishment of a dying patient's family. As the United States government tries to balance its Medicare budget the elderly will be expected to assume responsibility for a greater share of their health costs.

With the costs of delivery of care to any patient increasing, and with new Medicare laws that fix *all* physician fees for delivery of any services to the Medicare patient, most physicians will be forced into either cost-saving measures or will limit the number of Medicare patients they see. Hardest hit are those physicians delivering primary care to large Medicare practices. Their response is to see no new Medicare patients, decrease services to the Medicare population, or decrease total numbers of Medicare patients served. Thus, Medicare patients' access to quality primary care physicians might reasonably be expected to decrease. As such laws and social programs become more pervasive in our society, physicians, especially those newly licensed ones, may face economic disincentives to caring for the elderly.

THEORIES OF AGING

Many different theories have been developed to explain the biology of aging. In general, these can be broken down into two groups: stochastic and developmental/genetic. Stochastic theories suggest that the lifelong accumulation of environmental insults ultimately destroys the organism's cellular mechanisms and results in death of the organism. In such theories, environmental stresses such as radiation result in accumulated damage sufficient to kill the organism. In the "Error Theory" genetic material is replaced until an error catastrophe of replication occurs. Such an error results in the death of the organism. Although certain products of aging, such as the cell protein lipofuscin, accumulate with age, no evidence supports the concept that such accumulation significantly harms the organism.

The developmental/genetic theories suggest that the genetic material present at the creation of the organism has a built-in clock for development, maturation, aging, then death of the organism. Cellular and genetic mechanisms are invoked to explain such phenomena as that observed by Haflick: cells taken from short-lived animals such as mice can only divide a small number of times before they are no longer capable of division. Many more divisions occur in cells taken from the longest-lived animals such as Galapagos turtles, which are known to survive for hundreds of years. Thus, we see that the genetic material present at the birth of an organism must program the total number of potential replications for each cell over the life of the organism. Neuro-endocrine mechanisms alone have also been postulated as causing aging. Whether hormonal changes are the result or the cause of aging has yet to be clearly established. Aging itself is multifaceted and includes contributions from all of these mechanisms, to varying degrees in different organisms.

LIFE EXPECTANCY VERSUS LIFE SPAN

An important concept is the distinction between life span and life expectancy. Life span represents the maximum biological potential for age in a given organism. In man it is about 115 years of age. Claims of certain peoples to have lived about 150 years have generally been discounted by sophisticated scientific dating techniques that analyze such tissue samples as tooth scrapings. Life expectancy, on the other hand, is a statistical calculation based upon cross-sectional studies of a given population. Life expectancy is an average number derived from the population. It can vary and increase significantly in given societies with environmental changes such as the introduction of public sanitation, improved health, and nutrition.

Life expectancy in the United States has increased greatly and is approximately ninety years of age for women, less for men. Life expectancy information must be interpreted with caution because cross-sectional data tends to reflect the "cohort effect." An eighty-eight-year-old person has lived through the accumulated environmental effects since the turn of this century, as have all persons of similar age in our society. Children born today will live in a cohort that endures the accumulated effects of the end of this century and the beginning of the next. Thus, each cohort of a population endures a different pattern of environmental stresses. Studies based on cross-sectional averages, which determine life expectancy for each cohort, tend to overemphasize cohort environmental stresses.

More meaningful statements about the biological effects of aging are made through longitudinal studies of people as they age. Examples of these are the Baltimore and Duke longitudinal studies. Such studies take years to perform and have a high drop-out rate, both of subjects and investigators. It is generally easier, though less valid, to conduct cross-sectional studies on specific cohorts. Conclusions drawn from such cross-sectional data may then be generalized to all populations, with the reservations already mentioned. The main advantage of longitudinal studies is that primary aging processes are more likely to be separated from secondary aging processes. In other words, those changes due to aging alone can be separated from those changes secondary to various environmental and cohort effects.

A final concern regarding studies upon aging populations can be highlighted by our FDA drug-testing procedures. Long before drugs are tested on human populations they are introduced in animal trials. In preliminary studies, drugs are given to younger animals. The cost of drug trials in older animals is considerably greater as animal colonies have to be maintained and grown into senescence before such animals can be used in drug trials. The cost of raising a herd of rats into old age is considerably greater than the cost for maintenance of a much younger group of animals. The drug exposure history of older animals can be easily controlled. This is not the case with people. When introduced into clinical trials, healthy young patients on no other medicine are easier to recruit in tests than are their elderly counterparts. The likelihood of taking one or more prescriptions or over-the-counter drugs increases significantly with the age of the individuals studied. Drug trial experience is often based on large groups of young volunteers, and usually much smaller groups of older participants.

Similar concerns about differences between young and old can be raised when considering such things as nutritional requirements for the elderly or normal laboratory values for the elderly. Oftentimes so-called recommended or normal values for the elderly may be derived from younger populations and may not take into account such factors as the gradual decline in basal metabolic rate with age.

THE NONSPECIFIC NATURE OF THE PRESENTATION OF DISEASE

Normal aging occurs at different rates in different individuals. And even within a given individual, different organ systems may age at different rates. Aging populations tend to become more heterogeneous, and generalizations about such populations of heterogeneous individuals become much more difficult to make. The rate at which a given organ system loses its reserve strength often determines the manner in which stress of an illness might manifest itself. Furthermore, if the stress is caused by a disease occurring in an organ system with large reserve strengths, the *symptoms* of that disease might be attributed to a noninvolved organ system that happens to have the least reserve strength. This principle is best outlined by the following example:

CASE 1

An eighty-three-year-old woman with a long history of smoking and borderline lung function goes to her doctor with complaints of increased shortness of breath. Initial examination fails to reveal a source for her problem, but a careful laboratory exam suggests a urinary tract infection. Treatment of the urinary tract infection results in decreased complaints of shortness of breath.

As mentioned, despite the pulmonary presentation, the disease was located in the urinary tract in this woman. In general, disease in the elderly often presents itself in such atypical fashion. Some diseases such as those of the thyroid tend to have different typical presentations in the old, from their usual typical presentations in the young.

The nonspecific nature of the presentations of diseases is the rule for elderly patients. Symptoms of such nonspecific presentations may manifest in one or all of the following categories: (1) increased confusion, (2) urinary incontinence, (3) falls, (4) decreased appetite and weight loss, and (5) fever.

Many diseases can have silent presentations in the elderly. When the above symptom complexes are reviewed, oftentimes a history of one or more of them can be elicited prior to the recognition of an illness. Autopsy studies done on the elderly reveal that as many as one third to one half of the elderly undergoing autopsy have pathological signs of previous heart attacks. These heart attacks had occurred in the absence of a history of prior heart disease, or symptoms of prior heart disease. These heart attacks, though painless, may well have been associated with a period of one of the nonspecific symptoms listed above.

Appendicitis is another condition that can go unrecognized because of its paucity of symptoms, and its failure to behave like acute appendicitis in younger patients. Ruptured appendixes without any history other than perhaps vague abdominal discomfort are not unusual. Fever is oftentimes absent.

A physician treating elderly patients often requires skills beyond those acquired through medical practice on younger adults. Consider the difference between these two patients:

CASE 2

A nineteen-year-old, previously healthy college junior is seen with a cough, sputum production, fever of 102, and physical exam that suggests pneumonia.

CASE 3

An eighty-five-year-old, with long-standing rheumatoid arthritis, chronic heart failure, and recent hospitalization for hip fracture is brought to her physician because the family is concerned about many recent episodes of urinary incontinence without fever, cough, or other symptoms. During exam she is forgetful. The baseline exam shows no change in her arthritis or healed hip fracture. Cardiogram shows an old heart attack. A chest x-ray finally reveals a large pneumonia.

The two cases involve the same disease process of acute pneumonia. Each has a very different presentation. If, while treating the eighty-five-year-old patient, the physician fails to consider all of her problems, that physician might actually overlook a chronic disease uninvolved in the initial presentation of the pneumonia. Intravenous fluids, considered a standard therapy for pneumonia, might actually dangerously worsen her heart failure. Prolonged bed rest for the pneumonia might severely aggravate the rheumatoid joint stiffness resulting in a crippled, bedridden patient despite the clinical resolution of the pneumonia with antibiotics. Such cases serve to illustrate the myriad interrelated complexities in the care of the geriatric patients.

IATROGENIC DISEASE

Iatrogenesis, disease caused by the physician, also increases in the elderly population. This is due in part to the altered drug metabolism of the aging, but also due in part to the greater likelihood of multiple drug use for multiple chronic conditions. Geriatric outpatients less than seventy years of age use drugs from 1.6 different categories, and patients over eighty-four use drugs from 2.6 different categories. The likelihood of an adverse drug reaction increases as the total number of drugs consumed increases. Polypharmacy with its attendant risks of adverse drug interactions is most pronounced in the hospitalized and institutionalized elderly. As many as 2 percent of geriatric admissions to British hospitals have been attributed primarily to drug reactions, while drug reactions have been considered as a contributing factor in as many as 8 percent of admissons to British hospitals.

Drug noncompliance, a problem in all populations, is especially common in the elderly. Failure of elderly populations to comply with the physician's prescribed plan can be as high as 50 percent. Almost half of such errors have been deemed to have potentially serious consequences. Problems with drug prescribing are the most obvious types of iatrogenesis. Failure to recognize drug-induced side effects is not unusual. Also, drugs taken safely for years might not be readily suspected when new symptoms develop in an otherwise stable geriatric patient. Any drug, whether new or old, can cause unwanted side effects. When elderly patients present their physician with new complaints, a good first rule of thumb is to do a drug review and see if any other physician has added a new medicine. If not, then the last medicine prescribed by the treating physician might well be considered as a likely candidate for any new symptoms.

PHYSIOLOGICAL CHANGES WITH AGE

Many of the so-called normal changes of aging are less likely to occur in certain groups of people. Such groups include senior masters athletes—a group less likely to show common cardiovascular changes with age. So, too, many of the changes listed here may occur in lesser degrees in various super-healthy subgroups of elderly. Most of the changes that will be mentioned occur to some degree in everyone, and they might best be referred to as common physiological changes with age.

Body composition, posture, and overall cellular physiology change with age. A general increase in total body fat, and decrease in lean muscle mass, for instance, can profoundly affect the way that certain drugs are distributed in the body. Drugs that are distributed in body fats, such as anesthetics, may take a bit longer to act and may have unexpectedly prolonged duration of action because of their increased distribution in the body's increased fat.

Total body water decreases with age. Any drug that is distributed in the body's water will therefore be present in higher concentrations because the volume that that drug occupies is decreasing with age. Alcohol is an example of a drug that becomes more toxic per ounce because it distributes in body water and is therefore present in a higher concentration in an older individual.

Higher amounts of free, active drug may also be present in the blood because of either a decrease in normal binding of drugs to blood proteins or, in the case of polypharmacy, an increase in competition between different drugs for a fixed number of protein binding sites. Some drug detoxification systems in the liver show decreases in activity with aging, while other types of drug detoxification systems tend not to change at all. As expected, these changes increase the variability of dose responses to drugs for the elderly and tend to increase the likelihood of adverse drug reactions.

In geriatric patients some organ systems require greater concentrations of drug to exert their effect because of a decrease in the number of drug receptors. In the aged, other organ systems may require smaller amounts of drug because of increased activity of the drug at the receptor. Examples of each of these include: (1) Some cardiac medications are required in *higher* concentrations because of *decreases* in receptor sensitivity; and (2) because of different pain thresholds, the elderly often require smaller amounts of pain medicine than might be expected for their younger counterparts when each are given pain stimuli of equal intensity.

The kidney shows a gradual, progressive loss of function with age. These changes are due in part to changes in blood flow and also changes in function and number of functioning kidney units called nephrons. As nephrons "drop out," the other nephrons are more strained and become more likely to "drop out" themselves.

Some of the nervous-system changes with age include decreases in nerve conduction and brain speed of processing information, giving rise to the poorly understood concept that IQ decreases with age. Standard IQ tests rely upon performance on time-limited exams. Because of the aforementioned decreases in speed of processing, such tests generally show decreases in IQ with increasing age. In contrast to this, more global tests of information and recall, such as vocabulary and total knowledge, are not "timed" and indicate that throughout the life span there are steady increases in these two functions. It should also be noted that most intellectual functions show sharp declines for the last few years of life. Presumably this is due to the impact of whatever disease or illness might be causing the demise of the individual. Brain weight and numbers of cells do decrease with age. Total brain volume can be shown to decrease with age also.

Special x-rays such as the CAT scan, which gives a photograph of brain tissue inside the skull and measures the decreases in volume associated with age, do not predict in any fashion which patients might have dementing illness. In fact, there is poor correlation between brain volume and IQ in the elderly. To date, no single test, except possibly brain biopsy or autopsy, can clearly establish the exact cause of a dementing illness.

Decreases in brain neurotransmitters have been clearly correlated with age. For some regions of the brain, such as the substantia nigra, the selective loss of dopomenergic neurons forms the biochemical basis for Parkinson's disease. With Parkinson's disease the decrease in brain dopamine can be reversed with drugs that inhibit the breakdown of that neurotransmitter. Increase in dopamine can reverse the tremor, muscle rigidity, and slowness of movement seen in Parkinson's disease. The concept of altered neurotransmitter levels causing disease is highlighted by current studies that suggest that Alzheimer's disease is predominantly associated with decreases in brain acetylcholine levels. Marked decreases in the enzyme choline acetyl transferase are present in such brains.

Drugs with anticholinergic properties (such as over-the-counter cold remedies, antihistamines, and antidepressants) clearly worsen the cognitive abilities of demented patients. In fact, such anticholinergic agents, when administered to normal controls, can clearly be demonstrated to impair cognitive functioning. Even though many classes of brain neuro-transmitters tend to decrease with age, certain enzymes and neurotransmitters increase with age. Such is the case for the enzyme monoamine oxidase. Increases in this particular enzyme are associated with depression. Depression with aging can occur with very subtle symptoms and may respond to different medications than depression in the young, especially because of changes in monoamine oxidase levels. For this reason depressed elderly patients should be tried on monoamine oxidase inhibitors if other standard therapies have failed.

Decreases in pain and temperature sensation predispose the elderly to burns and accidents. Decreases in responses to changes in environmental stimuli, and decreases in such things as numbers of sweat glands, make older persons more prone to environmental changes that might result in heat stroke or hypothermia. Clearly, any drug, social factor, or disease that might further disturb a person's ability to sense or to regulate his/her body temperature increases the risk of either of these two illnesses, hypo- or hyperthermia.

Gastrointestinal changes with age include decreased stomach acid output, increased ph of stomach secretions, decreased gastric and colonic motility, and decreased absorption of some substances such as calcium and iron. Associations with these changes include minor alterations in drug absorption, pernicious anemia because of decreased absorption of Vitamin B_{12}, and osteoporosis—a bone disease aggravated by decreases in calcium absorption.

Cardiac changes with age include increases in conduction system abnormalities and increased calcification of the heart valves. There is noted an age-related decrease in the maximum exercise potential. Resting cardiac function stays fairly constant and normal with age. Despite the fact that cardiac conditions are listed as the leading cause of death of the elderly, few studies have been able to clearly document age-related decreases in the resting cardiac function.

Changes in pulmonary function include an increase in total lung volume but actual decreases in useful working lung tissue. In addition, because of changes in connective tissue and decreases in mucociliary clearance, the cough reflex becomes less effective and increases the susceptibility of the elderly to bronchopneumonia. Interestingly, it is the gradual decline in the lungs' ability to provide adequate ventilation for the body that most closely correlates with the biological potential for life span. On average, the age at which decreasing lung function no longer permits ventilation is about 115 years of age.

There is an increased frequency of many malignancies with age. Some malignancies are seen almost exclusively in the elderly, such as chronic lymphocytic leukemia. Decreases in both immune function and immune surveillance are thought to play a role in the development of many malignancies with aging. Also, because diseases such as tuberculosis were pandemic at the turn of the century, decreases in immune function can result in the reactivation of cases of tuberculosis that might have been quiescent for fifty years.

Changes in the special senses of hearing and vision have their own obvious contributions to the well-being of the elderly. High-frequency hearing loss (presbycusis) commonly occurs with aging, often accelerated by sound pollution. The most common visual change with aging is "far sightedness" (presbyopia). This results from a progressive stiffening of the lens of the eye, with the inability of the lens to focus on near objects. For this reason bifocals are often worn in order to see near objects while vision remains intact for far objects. Such decreases in auditory or visual abilities often increase a person's sense of isolation and both can contribute to disease states such as depression or pseudodementia. Pseudodementia is a state of apparent dementia, virtually indistinguishable from true dementia. However, the cognitive losses result from depression. Unlike dementing illness, pseudodementia resulting from depression can be reversed with the introduction of antidepressant medication.

Oftentimes, despite thorough clinical and laboratory evaluation of an apparent demented patient, a geriatrician will embark upon a trial of antidepressants because of the marked similarities between depression and dementia. It is indeed gratifying when the apparent demented patient improves and becomes normal on antidepressant medication. Studies of presumed demented patients have revealed that some patients' cognitive losses were not caused by dementia but rather were caused by sensory deprivation and/or depression. Similar observations can be made for the special sense of vision. Patients with marked visual losses can often appear to be demented when in fact their losses in abilities are not due to disease in the brain but rather due to disease in the eye.

Retinal illumination decreases significantly with age due to increases in lens opacity and decreases in resting pupil size. It is not unusual to restore a person's reading ability by increasing illumination—e.g., placing those patients in full sunlight. If the intensity of the lights in a person's environment is not steadily increased over time, age-related changes will cause a steady decrease in functional information reaching the retina. When visual testing is performed by optometrists, it is often done under ideal conditions with full illumination. Such visual tests may show "no changes" in visual acuity while patients continue to complain that their eyes just aren't any good and that the "doctor must be wrong." If the eye test had been performed under circumstances similar to the patients' environmental illumination, then the visual acuity might indeed have been much worse than under optimum conditions.

Smell, taste, and chewing ability all tend to change with age. Usually such changes can result in a decrease in the general level of nutrition. If someone is toothless, dentures must fit well in order to masticate food. The gums resorb steadily with age, and will change the fit of a pair of dentures over a period of time. Special diets may be prescribed for persons with diabetes or high blood pressure. Salt or sugar restrictions may render ordinary diets unpalatable. Of the four main taste sensations—bitter, acid, sweet, and salty—there is relatively greater loss of both sweet and salty taste sensations. Such losses may increase the tendency of elderly patients to over-salt or over-sweeten their food. All such changes are augmented by a concomitant decrease in the sense of smell. Also the wearing of dentures may further decrease one's ability to taste food.

All the special senses are vital to maximum functioning. Suffice it to say that weight loss, when seen in the elderly, is usually multifactoral and even after the usual endocrine, structural, and physiological diseases have been ruled out, the astute physician should be sure that proper oral/dental/special senses evaluations have been performed.

DISEASE CONSIDERATIONS WITH AGE

As noted earlier, some diseases have very different presentations in young cohorts versus older ones. Some diseases may be present in the elderly in such a fashion that they might mimic a different disease entirely. Other diseases such as Parkinson's and dementia seem to be unique to the aging population. A number of the most important will be mentioned here. Certain "conditions" not considered diseases per se, occur quite commonly in the aging population and will also be mentioned.

Such conditions might include "falls," social isolation, urinary incontinence, and decreased nutrition. Diseases with a unique predilection to the elderly are stroke, dementia, osteoporosis, debilitating rheumatologic disorders, and certain cancers, as well as endocrine and infectious diseases. More than half of the population over age sixty-five has some abnormality of cardiac function. Cardiac disease is the leading cause of death in the elderly. Progressive sclerosis of the fibrous structures in the heart and calcification of some of those structures can lead to heart rhythm problems, decreases in maximum movement of heart valves and heart muscle, and overall decrease in cardiac function. Athrosclerosis is a disease of blood lipids that results in depositing of cholesterol-laden plaques in blood vessel walls. These plaques limit the size of blood vessel lumens, and if severe enough, can even stop the flow of blood through a vessel. Athrosclerotic disease in the major blood vessels of the heart leads to "heart attacks"; This is a condition where part or all of the heart has a greater demand for blood than can be met by diseased blood vessels. The overloaded, undernourished muscle causes pain from too little blood (angina) or, if the overload is severe enough, the muscle dies resulting in myocardial infarction.

Hypertension is a multifactoral disease that becomes more prevalent with age. It can aggravate all forms of heart disease, predispose the patient to athrosclerosis, and aggravate many types of renal, neurologic, and opthalmologic diseases.

Stroke

Changes in blood vessels that might cause a heart attack by progressive occlusion, are not limited to that organ. Rather, these changes occur throughout the vascular beds of the body. One of the most devastating consequences of occlusion of blood vessels to the brain is stroke. When a blood vessel to the brain is occluded and if the surrounding vessels are unable to support the brain tissue, that tissue in the distribution of the affected blood vessel dies. Such losses are manifested by the signs and symptoms of acute massive brain loss, generally seen as the inability to properly move a limb or complete sophisticated activities such as speech or writing. With proper rehabilitation, training, and the passage of time, some brain deficits due to stroke can be overcome almost completely.

Preventive measures that slow the rate of progression of athrosclerosis clearly have a role in the prevention of both stroke and heart attack. Chief among these is lifelong blood pressure control. Limiting dietary cholesterol and fat intake, increasing dietary fiber, and daily exercise are also preventive measures for all forms of vascular disease. Of course avoidance of tobacco in all forms is also a major prophylaxis against athrosclerosis. Finally, new on the horizon are drugs that can lower the serum cholesterol or improve other of the blood lipids associated with athrosclerosis. Some agents such as aspirin can alter the properties of blood and make it much less able to deposit in blood vessels thus retarding the cholesterol plaques.

Hypertension

Changes in blood vessel walls, kidney function, and blood-pressure-sensing mechanisms all cause cuff readings of blood pressure to increase steadily with age. Elderly hypertensives may respond to different types of drugs than younger hypertensives. The need to decrease blood pressure to prevent multiple complications is no less important in the old than in the young. Unfortunately, because of the decreased sensitivity in the body's control mechanisms for regulating blood pressure, correction of blood pressure to acceptable lower levels may not be possible. Medications that lower blood pressure can also predispose the elderly to falls, especially if rapid changes in posture are encountered. Getting out of bed after resting in the lying position is one such posture change that can predispose to falls. A medication that lowers the blood pressure to "normal," might so delay the body's pressure-sensing mechanism that, immediately upon standing, the blood pressure might be too low, resulting in lightheadedness and possibly even a faint (syncope).

Arthritis

Complaints of aching joints or muscles may be signs of underlying arthritic disease. Diseases that result in decreased strength or decreased joint mobility all contribute to persons' decreased ability to move through their environment. Extreme cases can result in an inability to turn over in or to get out of bed without assistance. Less extreme might be the inability to climb three flights of stairs to the apartment that one has lived in for thirty years, progressive inability to get into a city bus, or in and out of a car.

Two major kinds of arthritis are osteoarthritis and rheumatoid arthritis. Both diseases can result in total joint destruction through different mechanisms. Rheumatoid arthritis is an autoimmune disease in which the joint lining (synovium) is progressively gobbled up by the patient's own blood cells for poorly understood reasons. In rheumatoid arthritis, pain and stiffness tend to be more pronounced in the morning. As joint destruction becomes more profound, stiffness and pain are more constant throughout the day. Modern orthopedic procedures allow replacement of some joints and can sometimes greatly increase the function of a limb or a joint.

Osteoarthritis is one of the most common conditions encountered with aging. Even in so-called "young-old" (those fifty-five to sixty-four years of age) the changes of this disease are present in over 80 percent of x-rays. The "wear and tear" of normal aging is thought to contribute to the degenerative nature of osteoarthritis. The gradual loss of the supple shock-absorbing qualities of normal bone and the biochemical failure to maintain the linings of joints result in a thinning of the joint cartilage and gradual reduction of joint spaces. Osteoarthritis, as with rheumatoid arthritis, is painful. But, unlike rheumatoid arthritis, the pain tends to increase over the course of the day. Destroyed joints of osteoarthritis can also be replaced using the same technology as for rheumatoid arthritis.

Of note, rheumatoid arthritis and osteoarthritis tend to have different patterns of joint involvement. Clinical distinction of the two diseases can be quite difficult if the disease process is seen at the time of total joint destruction. Nonsteroidal anti-inflammatory drugs (such as aspirin) and exercises to maintain muscle strength are quite important. These modalities must be balanced against their potential to increase joint destruction if exercise is too vigorous. Drugs that limit inflammation, such as the nonsteroidals already mentioned, can help to slow the progress of joint destruction and decrease the pain associated with many rheumatologic diseases. However, because of the side effects of such drugs and poor pain control, drug treatment of arthritis can be complex and unrewarding.

Endocrine Disease

The two most common disease groups found in the elderly are those of altered thyroid metabolism and those of altered sugar metabolism. Hypo- and hyperthyroidism occur more commonly with increased age. Certain types of hyperthyroidism seem unique to the elderly. A thyroid gland that produces too much thyroid hormone causes signs and symptoms of hypermetabolism such as heat intolerance, diarrhea, heart failure, weight loss, increased sweating, and eye muscle problems. The eye problems are much more common in elderly patients than their younger counterparts. Too low an output of thyroid hormone can cause hypothyroidism and symptoms of constipation, mental slowing, cold intolerance, weight gain, weakness, and also heart failure. Hyper- and hypothyroidism can both cause decreases in cognitive function indistinguishable from dementia.

Altered carbohydrate metabolism can result in diabetes. Signs of diabetes are attributable to the high blood sugars seen in this disease and include increased thirst, increased urination, nighttime urination, weight loss, and increased appetite. When diabetes occurs later in life it is likely to be responsive to dietary and oral medication management, rather than insulin. If the obese diabetic is unable to lose weight, however, insulin must often be initiated. Increases in body fat seen with age decrease the body's ability to handle dietary sugar. Long-standing diabetes can result in death from heart disease or disability from blindness, nerve damage, foot infection, subsequent amputation, or kidney failure. Diet and exercise are pillars of most diabetes treatment. Diabetes is the leading cause of blindness in the United States at this time and is also one of the most common diseases of the aged.

Osteoporosis

This disease costs billions of dollars annually and affects millions of Americans. No symptoms at all occur with this disease until the point that skeletal failure occurs and a fracture results. It is the major contributing factor to hip fracture in the elderly. The bones of a person with osteoporosis may appear quite normal under a microscope, but architecturally they lack all of the structural support they once had. Changes with age, aggravated by poor dietary habits, alcohol consumption, smoking, poor exercise habits, and a host of other factors cause normal bones to become thinner and thinner over time.

Osteoporosis results when the normal bone remodeling processes do not lay down as much bone as is being destroyed by normal processes. Contrary to popular belief, the bone is a very active metabolic structure. The imbalance between increased bone loss and inadequate bone deposition gradually (i.e., over thirty to forty years) results in weakened bones that fracture easily with trauma. Obviously the weaker the bone, the more likely a fracture will result from seemingly trivial trauma. Hips, spine, wrists, and the shoulder are the most often involved. Spine fractures result in a variety of back pain syndromes that can be perplexing. Over time such spinal fractures contribute to a decrease in the person's total height with age. They also result in the stooped back seen in the very old. Hormonal changes at menopause and the decreased skeletal mass of women uniquely predispose them to osteoporotic fractures at much younger ages than men.

Treatment programs for osteoporosis focus on reduction of risk factors, elimination of contributing illnesses, exercise, increased dietary calcium consumption, proper diet, and proper Vitamin D metabolism. Finally, estrogen replacement has been shown to be a safe and effective treatment for osteoporosis in postmenopausal women. Though once controversial, estrogen replacement is fast becoming a mainstay of modern treatment of osteoporosis in women. The drawback is that estrogen treatment can cause increases in postmenopausal bleeding and can even quickly unmask and aggravate previously unrecognized tumors of the uterus. All women should have routine gynecological evaluations, but any women on estrogen therapy *have* to have mandatory gynecological follow-ups.

Dementia

Dementia results from a number of diseases that cause progressive loss in all cognitive spheres. These include declines in function of memory, language, judgment, motor performance, and visuo-spatial skills. Also, concomitant with or even preceding these losses, changes in personality and behavior might be manifest, often with decreased social and occupational functioning. All of the above changes can be produced by *any* drug, at *any* time. Seemingly stable patients, on a given regimen for years might have drugs "overlooked" as a cause of an apparent dementing process. In the complex evaluation of dementing illness, complete drug cessation is attempted whenever possible. If the cognitive changes reverse with cessation of drugs, then a drug-induced delirium was the culprit, not a true dementia. Some clouding of level of consciousness is usually apparent when trying to distinguish delirium from dementia.

By far the most common cause of dementing illness is Alzheimer's disease. Other common causes include multi-infarct dementia resulting from multiple small strokes, and also pseudodementia. Pseudodementia was mentioned earlier and is the apparent dementia caused by depression. Cognitive losses resulting from depression can be quite gratifying to treat since they represent one of the truly reversible causes of dementia. Of note in the treatment of depression in the elderly is the important role of electroshock therapy. Though oftentimes scorned because of popular fear and misconception, electroconvulsive therapy is the fastest, safest, and probably the most effective modality for treatment of depression in the elderly.

Alzheimer's disease, when present, is a devastating illness: "the disease of the century." It has been said to "rob the mind of the patient and steal the soul of the family." Caring for such patients especially in their early wandering and disturbed stages can "be a 36-hour day." (See the book *36-Hour Day* for a practical discussion of life with Alzheimer's patients.) At the present time, between two and four million Americans and 5 percent of those over the age of sixty-five suffer from this illness.

Over one-half of the more than one million chronic care beds in this country are occupied by Alzheimer's patients. The cost of care for these patients is presently twelve billion dollars and is certain to increase. Despite the fact that no cure and few even mildly effective treatments are known at present, certain parallels between this disease and Parkinson's disease suggest pharmacological approaches to the management of the Alzheimer's patient. Furthermore, application of proper principles of geriatric medicine to such patients can significantly improve their functional status. Drug side effects, concurrent medical illnesses, problem behaviors, and failing family supports, when recognized and properly addressed, can keep the Alzheimer's patient in the community and out of both hospital and long-term care arenas. This allows such patients to receive care from people they once knew and with whom they may still have some rapport. Such rapport can greatly diminish the need for psychotropic or physical means of restraint of such patients.

Incontinence

Incontinence of either urine or stool can be embarrassing, lead to social isolation, and when coupled with debility and/or skin wounds, can lead to profound decreases in ability to maintain hygiene. Such decreases in hygiene lead to further isolation and increase the chances of suffering a serious infection. Incontinence may be defined as the involuntary, accidental leakage of urine from the bladder. Such accidents can be large or small and obviously may have different precipitating causes. Flow sheets of types (i.e., large versus small) of accidents, frequency of accidents, and precipitating causes of accidents greatly aid the geriatrician in assessing response to different modalities. They also may aid in diagnosis of the type of incontinence. Such flow sheets are difficult to maintain properly. In the home setting, the patient or caregiver must be willing and able to maintain such a diary. In the institutional setting, staffing patterns must be sufficiently ample to allow for careful individual attention to such seemingly hopeless problems as incontinence.

Incontinence is often one of the "silent" problems of aging. If accidents occur infrequently, or the patient has developed a socially acceptable method of hiding the problem, then relatives, acquaintances, and even physicians can be completely unaware of the silent problem of incontinence. Prevalence of urinary incontinence problems in community-dwelling geriatric populations has been estimated at 30 percent. This figure increases to about 50 percent for hospitalized elderly patients. Studies have suggested that physicians recognize less than 10 percent of incontinence in hospitalized patients and attempt to manage but a small fraction of that population. The great majority of incontinent patients go both unrecognized and unassessed or untreated. Problems such as incontinence involve *all* of the complex principles of geriatric medicine outlined in this chapter. A proper approach to such problems highlights the importance of the unique skills of a geriatric specialist and the unique management of such problems.

The duration of the symptoms of incontinence determines what approach should be used by the caregiver. New onset or transient incontinence *should be reversible* if properly assessed and managed. Too often the new onset of incontinence is viewed as a necessary part of aging and management strategies are developed for the patient that do nothing to reverse the incontinency. Use of incontinence pads is an example of a treatment for incontinence that does little to reverse the problem. Incontinence when long-standing is much more difficult to assess and to treat, though a large number of these can also be reversed. Reversible causes of transient incontinence include such precipitators as urinary tract infections, diuretics, fecal impaction, decreased mobility from concurrent illness, transient confusion from drugs, etc. Of course, all of the above can be superimposed upon causes for long-standing incontinence, which can be due to multiple causes. With the flow sheets mentioned previously, assessment of therapies for multifactoral incontinence can be attempted. Long-standing, established incontinence is caused by one or all of the following factors:

Stress Incontinence

Weakness of the pelvic floor or urinary sphincter muscle causes urine to leak when abdominal pressure is increased as with a cough or a sneeze. Pelvic floor exercises or medicines that increase the sphincter tone can reverse this type of incontinence.

Urge Incontinence

Patients suddenly sense the urge to urinate and shortly thereafter lose their urine. Disordered synchronization of bladder contraction and urine release cause such problems. This type of incontinence may respond to drugs that improve the synchronization of the bladder and the urinary sphincter.

Overflow Incontinence

Obstruction to the urine outflow, as with urinary tumors, increased prostatic size in males, or pressure from rectal tumors or stool, causes the urine to build up and results in a steady dribbling of urine around the obstruction in an uncontrolled fashion. Treatment of overflow incontinence centers around removal of the obstruction. This may be as simple as an enema or as complex as the major reconstructive surgery of the lower genito-urinary tract. In males, removal of part or all of the prostate gland can eliminate this form of incontinence.

Functional Incontinence

The final, and perhaps most common and under-recognized form of incontinence is *functional* incontinence. Such patients are incontinent as a function of some other reason that prevents them from getting to the bathroom in time. In the case of a bedridden fracture patient, it is easy to understand functional incontinence. In the case of an arthritic who has difficulty getting out of a chair and is unable to ambulate until "limbered up," such functional incontinence might be harder to recognize. The fracture patient should resolve his incontinence when the fracture is healed and he has returned to normal mobility. The arthritic patient may need an anti-inflammatory drug before being able to get to the bathroom. Or the arthritic, if unable to tolerate the imflammatory medication, might become continent if given a commode chair in the same room instead of having to walk down the hall and up a flight of stairs to get to the bathroom. A urinal can also result in continency in such a patient.

Such approaches to problem solving are very functionally oriented and nonmedical. In fact, they extend the medical assessment and functionally tailor treatment programs to the patient. Such treatments can be very rewarding and can greatly improve the functional status and quality of life for the patient. In the case of incontinence, such treatments prevent social isolation and greatly reduce the likelihood of institutionalization.

Social Isolation

Social isolation can easily result from the death of a spouse, especially if that spouse was at a higher functional level, or possibly did all the driving or even just helped the patient up and down the front steps. The death of one spouse is often followed within a few months by the death of the other spouse. Reasons such as those mentioned might be equal to or possibly even more important than grief, predisposing the remaining spouse to decreased mobility and death. Changes in family mobility and structure in our society often place children in cities different from their aging parents. Many children are themselves sixty years old with their own health problems, and these problems might preclude them from caring for an ailing eighty-year-old parent. Friends and social contacts of an eighty-year-old are likely to have either died or suffered from health problems that might limit their ability to help. Shopping, easily performed when these people were in the late forties and fifties, might pose a tremendous obstacle to someone in their eighties or nineties. The inability to get out leads to social isolation and increases dependency upon others for support. All too often, hospital admission or disease episodes are precipitated by failure of informal support systems to support the socially isolated frail elderly.

Falls

Falls occur quite frequently in the elderly population and have many predisposing factors. Falls are the major cause of accidental death in the elderly population, and are one of the ten leading causes of death in the population over age sixty-five. Although many falls can be due to slips and trips, a number are associated with chronic and acute diseases. So, too, medications can increase the tendency to fall, either by causing lightheadedness or by causing changes in the body's balance mechanisms. Decreases in visual abilities can cause patients to misjudge the steps and to trip over things because they didn't see them. Also, as people age, they tend not to pick up their feet high enough off the ground. Because of this, seemingly unimportant obstructions on the floor can result in trips in the home environment. If the patient has a hard floor in one room and a thick pile rug in another room, it is only a question of time before the patient starts to trip on the thick pile rug. Loose throw rugs are also associated with.falls. Poor lighting, and unsafe railings or unsafe bathrooms are notorious for causing falls among the elderly. Poor footwear and improper use of assistive devices such as canes or walkers can also result in falls. In institutions, many falls occur out of the wheelchair.

It is the task of the geriatric careprovider to assess the safety of the home or institutional environment in addition to identifying disease processes that might contribute to falls. So, too, the caregiver must be constantly aware of the impact of medication upon balance in the elderly. Polypharmacy and adverse drug effects must constantly be guarded against.

FOR DISCUSSION

In this chapter basic theories of aging, physiology of aging, and management of common medical conditions of the aged have been outlined. The following exercise will further enhance your understanding of the complex, interrelated problems of aging.

First, imagine that you have lived in the same dwelling for forty years. Then, for each condition below, imagine performing the activity listed. Imagine groups of conditions and groups of activities. Discuss the differences.

CONDITIONS	ACTIVITIES
- new onset heart failure that limits your exercise tolerance to the point that you cannot climb more than three stairs - losing your useful vision - losing your useful hearing - tending a bedridden spouse - recent stroke that prevents you from speaking - right foot amputation - broken hip - no income except $300 social security per month - new onset of incontinence - living in a long-term care facility - being confined to a wheelchair	- driving - going to the second-floor bathroom - climbing to a fourth-floor apartment - lighting the furnace for the winter - going to the drug store for a new prescription - the pharmacist tells you the medicine will cost $100 per month - grocery shopping - using the telephone - visiting your best friend across the road - walking across a crowded parking lot - parking in a parking garage to get x-rays taken at the local health complex - seeing your children over the holidays, especially if they live in another city - going to a restaurant in daytime, or at night - seeing a doctor who is located forty miles from your dwelling - walking outside on uneven ground in winter - stepping off a curb

REFERENCES

Andres, R., Bierman, E. C., Hazzard, W. R. (eds.). *Principles of Geriatric Medicine.* New York: McGraw-Hill Inc. 1985; basic science of aging and disease processes.

Calkins, E., Davis, P. J., Ford, A. B. (eds.). *The Practice of Geriatrics.* Philadelphia: W. B. Saunders, 1986; practical approach to medical problems of aging.

Exton-Smith, A. M., Weksler, M. E. (eds.). *Practical Geriatric Medicine.* Edinburgh: Churchill Livingstone Inc., 1985; disease-related approach to aging with excellent sections on general and societal considerations.

Kenney, R. A. *Physiology of Aging—A Synopsis.* New York: Yearbook Medical Publishers 1982; easiest to read most concise book on this subject.

Libow, L. S., Sherman, F. T. (eds.). *The Core of Geriatric Medicine— A Guide for Students and Practitioner.* St. Louis: C. V. Moby Company, 1981; basic approaches outlined with good discussion of special senses.

Mace, M. L., Rabins, P. V. *The 36-Hour Day.* Baltimore: Johns Hopkins University Press, 1981; a practical guide for families of demented patients.

Milne, J. S. *Clinical Effects of Aging—A Longitudinal Study.* New Hampshire: Croom Helm, 1985; a very well designed longitudinal study, with excellent discussion of problems in study design.

5

The Elderly and Their Environment

Marian Deutschman

What is the environment? It's that area "outside our skin" (Lawton 1988). It can be defined as the total surrounding context for a person, including a combination of many forces, among them physical, social, structural, and economic. It can include the geographic location, the technological surroundings, the social environment, and the culture.

The physical environment includes temperature, light, physical objects, furniture, sensory materials, personal space, territory, buildings, sites, spaces, and the relationships of all these features. Norms represent the social environment—how the users of the space are expected to behave in that physical space. The culture in which the person is located affects the development of the physical environment through assumptions handed down over the years (Steele 1973). In an organization, culture represents "the way we do things around here" (Deal & Kennedy 1982).

Do people control the environment or does the environment control people? That's an unresolved problem. However, when a person is elderly and sensory deficient or disabled, the individual is more vulnerable to a poor fit between the environment and her needs. On the positive side, that same elderly individual may benefit from even a small change in the physical space.

Recognition that the physical environment can facilitate or hinder the behavior of its users opens up a whole array of possibilities for changes in the functioning of an organization or an individual. Knowledge of the relationship of behavior and environment offers opportunities for strategic change, therapeutic change, and creative change.

THE THEORY

There are at least three ways in which the physical environment may be uniquely significant to people as they grow older: (1) the environment may influence normal levels of functioning, (2) it may compensate for reduced mobility, and (3) it may accelerate the onset of impairments and shape the experience of disability (Hiatt 1982).

The physical setting and artifacts intruding into this setting can act as moderators, facilitators, or inhibitors of behavior. Settings should not be viewed as "sacred" and unchangeable but as opportunities for evolving, experimenting, and expanding options.

A person acts in accordance with what an environment expects of her (Pastalan 1980). Lawton and Nahemow (1973) argue that no person is immune to the seductive power of the easy life. There is no question that it is possible to discourage independent behavior in the name of service to the elderly. Tobin & Lieberman (1976) conclude that "an environment that does not encourage full use of potential may cause irreversible deterioration."

As an elderly person's needs and capabilities change, adaptive strategies are required to move toward a better fit between the person and the environment, either in a different setting or by providing choices or adjustments in the present environment. Although there are individual differences, in areas where an older individual has experienced changes in needs and preferences, she may be especially vulnerable to environmental incongruence (Kahana, Liang & Felton 1980).

For example, when a person who can no longer delay gratification is placed in an environment where a great deal of delay is expected, problems result (Kahana et al. 1980). Certain behaviors that appear to others as uncooperative or belligerent, and which may be destructive to the patient's physical health as well, may be serving to counteract the individual's feelings of powerlessness and low self-esteem (Nelson & Farberow 1980). Some Alzheimer patients have been found to do better with a roommate (bonding relationships). Materials for simple activities to incorporate a patient's interests and lifestyle into the daily care routine provide a stabilizing influence (Greene 1986). Agitation, which is common in these patients, can worsen if they are restricted from expending their high level of energy. Competence does not rest exclusively in the person but in the relationship between the person and the surroundings she is trying to manipulate (Steinfeld 1979).

The congruence model proposes that individuals are most likely to be found in environments congruent with their needs. Dissonance between the fit and the need leads to the individual leaving in a free-choice situation. Stress occurs when choice is unavailable or when an individual must continue to function in an inappropriate environment (Stern 1970; Zimring 1981).

Nehrke (1984, 1983, 1981) proposes that the impact of incongruence would vary according to the importance of the dimension to the individual. The more important the dimension, the more likely incongruity on that dimension would motivate the individual to leave the environment and seek a situation where person-environment fit can be achieved. In Nehrke's studies in long-term care, the dimensions demonstrating the highest levels of incongruence at all times of testing were "responsive health care," "lack of respect from staff," and "social stimulation." Increasing the level of congruence within these three dimensions would, theoretically, increase the probability of the occurrence of well-being.

The environmental docility hypothesis proposes that the importance of the environment, as a determinant of behavior, increases as competence decreases (Lawton 1975; Lawton & Simon 1968). Environmental constraints or facilitators matter more (not less, as might be assumed) to the more impaired older individual.

Lawton's "Press Competence Model and the Older Person as Active Initiator" states that the more competent one is, the more objectionable an environment is when it lacks stimulation. A mild increase is pleasurable. Problem-solving situations, an increment above one's present capabilities, becomes learning. Many programs that are designed to reduce environmental pressure for the institutionalized elderly produce negative consequences and a drop in competence. It's important to provide an increase in environmental pressure that avoids repeated failures—a deterrent to learning. When a person is in a zone of maximum comfort, the potential for adaptive behavior is increased (Lawton 1970). Individualized change or restructuring can provide this therapeutic potential if an elderly person is evaluated not only from the traditional biological-organic approach but from a psychosocial perspective that includes his or her individual coping ability.

Continuing ties with preferred members of one's social network, personal responsibilities, and social need gratification appear to have the greatest importance in determining elderly morale and life satisfaction (Harel 1981). Even a bedridden patient has an innate drive to interact with, manipulate, and master the environment (Brink 1979). There are suggestions that much of the behavior commonly referred to as senility can be produced by depriving the long-term patient of problem-solving activities (Brink 1979).

Choice is a crucial variable in providing a sense of control. Exercise of choice, even when inconsequential, can have psychological consequences of increased confidence (Langer 1975). Health-care staff and caregivers tend to see themselves as the predominant decison makers. A study by Ryden (1985) indicated caregivers, at home or in institutions, do not emphasize the availability of options to the elderly.

The degree to which the elderly person focuses on the past may be a function of the environment. As an individual's activity space becomes restricted, the past, through reminiscence, may become the source of environmental experiences (Strauss, Aldrich & Lipman 1976).

THE SENSORY ENVIRONMENT

Aging brings with it normal changes in sensory efficiency. For example, the lens in the eye thickens and yellows resulting in a change in the perception of close values (lightness or darkness) of color. Muscles controlling pupil dilation are weaker, requiring three times more light than that needed by younger people. Tolerance to glare and reflections is decreased. Problems with depth perception and color differentiation require an objective assessment of the physical environment to accommodate these changes. If distortions are to be avoided, wall coverings that are reflective or wall patterns that are disturbing must be evaluated from the perspective of the person who is confined to a space for long periods of time. The selective use of color can minimize the adverse effects of sensory deprivation while enhancing mood. These choices should be based on the space available (darker colors make the room appear smaller), on the preferences of the users ("peachy" colors seem to add warmth to a room and are well received), and on the color of other items in the room (the need to coordinate and harmonize). There are some color research conclusions that can be used as guidelines (e.g., warm colors are known to enhance appetite) but it must be kept in mind that wall colors are only a backdrop for the activity of users who bring their own colors into the space. Color-coding or cueing can be recommended to improve function, but it should be based on the solution of a specific problem. Increased lighting can assist performance of the activities of daily living (Cooper, Gowland & McIntosh 1986).

The sounds of a typical home and a typical long-term health care facility are quite different. Until these sounds are isolated by taping them or by closing one's eyes and listening, one may be unaware of the auditory disturbances that may overwhelm a dementia patient, for example. These sounds may also be a source of stress to the caregivers. Extended observation of activity in one nursing home solarium resulted in a headache because the stereo and television were on at the same time. This created a disturbing, unspecific noise. No staff member stayed in the room long enough to sense this (Deutschman 1980). Unnecessary sounds can be eliminated or modified, but first they must be identified by taking the time to do so. Sound absorbent materials on walls and floors, and window treatment can reduce the irritation. The elderly often have more difficulty hearing high-frequency sound and higher-register voices. Shouting may only increase the difficulty.

The sense of touch can be used as a support to replace other sensory deficiencies. Textures can be used as landmarks for finding one's way in the physical space. Cold, hard, reflective surfaces can be replaced with more diversity in textures. Care should be taken when making changes so that the elderly person's system of landmarks remains intact.

Within most cultures, rules and meanings of touch are different for men and women. In a recently reported study, a psychologist arranged for a group of nonelderly patients, who were about to undergo major surgery, to be touched by a nurse in the following way: the nurse came in to tell each person about the operation and the aftercare, and in doing touched the patient twice briefly, once on the hand for a few seconds, and again on the arm for a full minute, and then as she was leaving she shook each person's hand. Women had strikingly positive reactions, lowering their blood pressure and anxiety both before surgery and for over an hour afterward. For men, both their blood pressure and anxiety rose and stayed elevated in response to being touched. It was suggested that strikingly different responses may occur because men in the United States find it harder to acknowledge dependency and fear than do women. A well-intentioned touch may be a threatening reminder of their vulnerability (Thayer 1988). Whether or not one can generalize from this study, differences in age, gender, and culture are worth noting when discussing the effects of touch.

Sulfide stain resistant fabrics may provide a necessary precaution for damage to furniture coverings by incontinence. Avoid using pads under carpeting, especially if a wheelchair or walker is used. Pads add a cushion under foot for those of us who have no problem with mobility, but hinder movement for those with ambulation difficulties. Avoid selecting irregular floor surfaces that are likely to be perceived as a hazard by the elderly. The Kellogg International Work Group on the Prevention of Falls by the Elderly (1987) reports that the prevalence of falls appears to involve roughly one-third of persons aged sixty-five and older. The fear of falling results in the floor being used for visual cues and floor surfaces become an especially significant factor in mobility. Highly waxed floor surfaces may be perceived as wet. Irregular floor surfaces such as brick, or even a simulated irregularity in floor tiles, can reduce mobility because of this fear of falling.

The importance of the sense of taste is evident in the tendency for the elderly to be preoccupied with detailed accounts of meals. These meals should be served to encourage self-feeding and to accommodate sensory needs as well as dietary restrictions. Color and texture play a significant role in enhancing appetite and in providing clear identification of different foods for those with visual deficiency.

Smell is used as a method by which a health-care facility is judged by outsiders. The odor of incontinence is unpleasant for both insiders and outsiders and should not be evident in a good facility. Pleasant odors can be used for reality orientation, reminiscence, and as a cue to appropriate behavior. The fresh smell of coffee, flowers, freshly baked bread or cookies, and other common smells of home can be restored to any setting with a little creativity.

NONVERBAL COMMUNICATION

Society's institutions establish, prescribe, and control nonverbal communication. "Nonverbal behavior in organizations is not limited to cues from bodily behavior, facial expressions, and voice transmission of messages. Territory and space, time, the building, a room, the seating design, artifacts and objects, exert environmental/behavioral influences" (Goldhaber 1983).

Appearance helps people form impressions of each other. In a health-care setting, staff expectations of patients/residents and subsequent communication are often based on appearance. Expectations influence the behavior of both the patients and staff in a reciprocal process. Aspects of appearance affect one person's influence over another. Physical appearance and attire signal status and approachability, and define context and role behavior. Institutional uniforms symbolically express status, therefore according the wearers more privacy and deference from others. Clothing indirectly determines social accessibility and directly communicates approachability (Burgoon 1982).

Attractiveness, status indicators, similarity of appearance, and signs of expertise affect the ability to persuade others. Facial expressions and tone of voice can accurately inform us of another's emotional state. Rosenthal (1979) found that physicians who were good encoders of vocal tones and facial expressions had more satisfied patients. Learning to recognize the importance of nonverbal behavior and its role in communication should be part of staff training in a health-care setting. However, the overriding conclusion that has emerged is that no simple generalizations about usage can be made for any particular nonverbal behavior. Consistent but highly specialized patterns are evident according to setting, nature of encounters, cultural, sociological, and personality characteristics.

Territory represents fixed-feature space while personal space moves with an individual. Hall (1973) suggests a basic difference in the manner in which different cultures use space. High-status personnel in an American organization, for example, usually have greater territory, protect their territory better, and invade the territory of lower status personnel (Goldhaber 1983). How much status does an institutionalized resident possess when a lifetime of accumulation of personal status is reduced to fit into the personal space/territory of a shared room in a nursing home, the size of which is dictated by building costs and government regulation? Minimum requirements usually become maximum requirements.

Definition of territories is a means of regulating social interaction, creating a sense of personal identity, promoting group identity/bonding, and warding off physical intrusions. In health-care settings, invasion of privacy into the personal space or territory of patients is commonplace.

Intrusions into others' territories or personal spaces may psychologically intimidate and signal dominance. Greenberg and Firestone (1977) and Sundstrom (1975) found that in response to increased surveillance, spatial intrusions, or psychological intrusions, people reduce self-disclosure and use more role-playing. When privacy is insufficient, the elderly may communicate their need through behaviors that include stress, retreat, withdrawal, setting up more territorial markers, and augmenting space if possible.

Furnishings and artifacts mark territories. Patterson (1978), in a study of territorial behavior among the elderly, found that the use of such territorial markers as "no trespassing" signs, welcome mats, and external surveillance devices reduced an elderly person's fear of property loss and personal assault. The more personalized the environment, the more the individual expresses uniqueness and autonomy. Decorations may reveal a person's sense of comfort and identification with an environment. Arrangement of furniture signals whether social encounters are permissible and expected.

To be alone when one wishes companionship can be as detrimental as the lack of privacy (Westin 1967). Kayser-Jones (1986) suggested that open-ward accommodations are a supportive environment for the elderly with functional and social losses.

Settings can have an effect on the values people place on themselves. Diversity of stimulation can trigger new perceptions, new connections of thoughts and feelings. In order for new patterns to emerge, a person must, of course, use the opportunities available. Sometimes individuals with a low self-worth accept inadequate settings as evidence of what they think they deserve.

THE ELDERLY IN THE HOME ENVIRONMENT

Safety and security are a prime concern, especially when the home of the elderly person is in an urban area. Some recommendations have already been suggested. Because falls are the leading cause of accidents, stairs and walkways should be clutter free. Handrails should be installed on both sides of stairs or on the right side for right-side dominant people. Appropriateness of the shoes, and especially their soles, is a safety consideration. Some soles may be too sticky or slippery and may need to be roughened with coarse sandpaper. Backless slippers are a hazard and should be avoided. Rugs, runners, and floor coverings should have a rubberized back to prevent curling and sliding. Rugs should never be used at the top or bottom of stairs. Double-faced tape can be used on the back of rugs to prevent skidding. Spills should be wiped up promptly to prevent falls.

Lamp switches should be easy to use and within easy reach. Electrical cords should be placed along the base of the wall and taped in place. When in doubt, don't use more than a 60-watt bulb, otherwise potential fires may melt the lampshade. Be sure grab-bars are installed and attached to the structural supports, especially in the bathroom. The tub area can be a potential hazard. A nonskid mat in the tub can reduce the risk significantly. A tub seat with adjustable legs may be appropriate. A raised toilet seat with rear locking brackets may provide necessary assistance. A hand-held shower can be attached to the faucet in the tub or sink. Skin integrity changes with aging, so hot water should be controlled to avoid scalding. Room heaters need screens for safety. The path from the bedroom to the bathroom should be well lighted. A phone should be installed at the bedside. An emergency exit plan should be prepared, rehearsed, and reviewed periodically.

Optimum storage in the kitchen should be located within comfortable reach. Reaching into high cupboard storage space can disturb the equilibrium of the elderly and result in a fall. A step stool with a handrail can assist reaching for high items if absolutely necessary. Avoid using unreliable ladders. Someone should be there to hold even the most reliable ladder.

Food and cleaning agents should never be stored in one cupboard area, thus avoiding the possibility of a mix-up and accidental poisoning. Medicines should be properly labeled, and should be thrown away when expired. Prominent visual cues in color should mark those medicines that are designed for external use only.

There are many adaptive devices occupational therapists can suggest to accommodate sensory deficiencies and restricted mobility. Objects with long handles can assist the elderly person with restricted movement to continue to perform the activities of daily living independently. Long-handled brushes and combs, dressing sticks, extended shoe horns, button hooks, zipper pulls, one-handed can openers, specially designed cutting boards, trigger-action squeezer reachers, long-handled sponges, Velcro closures, and nonskid material such as suction cups provide low-cost supports. Door knob adapters permit arthritic hands to better manipulate door opening. Magnifying glasses, large number dials for the telephone, talking books, talking clocks, and a whole array of visual aids are available through low vision centers in many cities, often in connection with the Association for the Blind.

The room temperature should never be set below 65 degrees. Concern over hypothermia or lowered body temperature has created an awareness for proper attire for the cold months. A handy cane device to assist those walking in cold, icy climates has an ice tip that snaps up and down when needed for stability. Many of these products can be found in medical health supply stores.

THE ELDERLY IN THE LONG-TERM CARE ENVIRONMENT

The pattern of illness and disease has changed in the past eighty years from predominantly acute conditions at the turn of the century to chronic conditions that are now the most prevalent health problem for elderly persons. The elderly are the heaviest users of health services, accounting for one-third of the country's personal health-care expenditures, even though they constitute only 12 percent of the population. Health-care utilization is also greatest in the last year of life and among the "old-old" individuals, those seventy-five or older.

By the turn of the century, half of the elderly population is expected to be sixty-five to seventy-four and half will be seventy-five or older. Life expectancy at age eighty-five has increased 24 percent since 1960 and is projected to increase another 44 percent by 2040. More people are surviving into their tenth and eleventh decades. This is significant for long-term care because both males and females eighty-five and older are four times more likely to be disabled than those sixty-five to seventy-four. Administration on Aging figures indicate that the number of aged individuals with significant difficulties in carrying out some or all the functions of daily living is growing by about 100,000 per year (Aging America 1986).

In 1985, an estimated 1.5 million persons resided in nursing homes. Although, at any given time, the proportion of institutionalized elderly in the elderly population has not changed significantly from the current 5 percent, the mean age at the time of institutionalization is expected to be higher and the level of abilities and skills of the institutionalized residents is likely to be lower. One in four will need long-term care assistance at some time during their later years. The greatest growth in nursing facilities is expected in the next two decades.

Resource Utilization Groups (RUGs) present a relatively new attempt at health-care cost containment. This new *prospective* payment system provides incentives for nursing homes to care for patients who require a higher level of the home's resources. The expected benefits of the RUGs system include easier access to nursing home care for patients requiring heavy or complex care, and more attention given to intensive rehabilitation of some patients.

Health-care practitioners have standardized skills and knowledge that they acquired off-site in preparation for the hospital setting. They are now attempting to apply these skills and knowledge to long-term care, which often results in role conflict and role ambiguity. When the medical culture of the acute care facility is carried over into long-term care, staff reinforce the medical milieu and the "patient" role. Both patient and staff are predisposed to activate the "sick patient" role. Staff respond to disruptive behavior with medication, restriction, and/or avoidance. Reciprocally, staff expect "good," "dependent," "nonacting out" behavior (Nicholson 1982). Staff role transition must take on a perspective that perceives physical and psychosocial care as equal in importance to the well-being of the individual (Nicholson 1982). Many of the problems faced by the elderly in receiving health-care services are related to problems in health-care communication between the health-care provider and the patient, as well as between members of the health-care team (Kreps 1984). Staff initiate and terminate by far the greater proportion of interaction with residents.

Solomon (1983) suggests that an unbalanced relationship exists between the staff member and the patient: "In the interactions between health care providers and elderly patients, interpersonal distance increases because of contingencies inherent in the sick and healer roles and disparities of status. These disparities include education, age roles, and real helplessness. The disparity in the distribution of power in the relationship increases the chance of capricious behavior on the part of the provider. Response-outcome may then become independent of behavior."

Stein, Linn, and Stein (1986) found that after three months in an institution there is evidence that the resident is beginning to accommodate to the environment. After only a short time in the nursing homes, residents are capable of "sizing up" the situation in accordance with outside "expert" opinion. Time does not seem to modify these perceptions. Perhaps that is because time alone cannot change the environment. It is well known that poorly trained staff (particularly aides who provide the bulk of care), high staff turnover, low wages, low morale, and the demands of the job all can contribute to a nursing home environment that is stressful for both patients and staff (Proch 1983). And yet, the nursing home is truly an end-stage home for most people who are admitted with a negative prognosis.

Harel (1981) suggests that nursing homes establish departments of resident services that would assess residents' preferences, identify and represent residents' psychosocial needs, and help formulate and coordinate care plans best suited to the specific needs of each resident. Unfortunately, institutional environments are generally not designed to be optimal environments for particular individuals, but more likely they attempt to serve the varying needs of heterogeneous populations.

Dependency is the result of an interplay between social contingencies and the biological vulnerability of the elderly (Baltes 1985). Some of the negative consequences of aging may be retarded or reversed by returning to the aged the right to make decisions, which can result in a feeling of competence.

Stress is an important issue to study when trying to understand the well-being of the elderly. The environment has the potential for intervention to enhance coping and thereby reduce stress. Negative life events are noxious only if one cannot cope. Coping depends on whether a situation is negatively appraised. Residual effects of external events differ according to individual differences (Kahana 1988). There are two opinions regarding the effects of stress. The stress-inoculation concept suggests that an abundance of early stress prepares persons by strengthening them for later stress. Another perspective suggests extended stress creates an increase in vulnerability. As mentioned earlier, environmental stressors represent the environmental incongruence requiring change in the person or in the environment. Some stressors have an impact on mental health, while others influence physical health; life frustrations can affect both; macro-events may influence neither. Institutionalization itself may not be as extremely stressful as once thought. Stress may be dependent on assumptions when entering, especially if there is significant rehabilitation potential. Older people have been found to be quite resilient and pro-active (Kahana 1988).

ENVIRONMENTAL COMPETENCE

Environmental competence has been defined as the degree to which individuals are aware of their physical facilities and are able to make decisions to provide a better fit between themselves and their settings (Steele 1973). Training in environmental competence can help individuals to identify their own needs and the needs of those in their care. Sometimes it may be necessary for a caregiver to assume a role of mediator between those who are less competent and what is often a rigid institutional environment or a home environment that is no longer appropriately meeting the needs of its users. This does *not* mean that the elderly person's wishes are ignored.

How does an individual develop environmental competence? Such competence involves the development of sensitivity; empathy and objectivity; taking into consideration the site, the building, the spaces (territories) with which a person, group, or organization is associated; the settings (collection of things surrounding a person physically and providing him/her with sensory stimulation); the arrangement and relationships of parts; properties of things (color, textures); consequences (comfort, visibility, moods evoked, memories triggered, ease/difficulty of performing activities, contacts, and stimulation). Though objectivity, empathy, and sensitivity overlap to some degree, each can be reviewed separately (Deutschman 1985). This process can be used to assess home environments as well as institutional settings.

Objectivity

The environment is often taken for granted and no longer critically viewed. After a relatively short period of time, even though the spaces may be used almost every day, they are no longer perceived objectively. Objectivity regarding physical space can start with an assessment of whether communication would be different if furniture were rearranged. Would the result be more privacy, fewer interruptions, and fewer distractions? Would a barrier at eye level provide more privacy? Barriers can be created with furniture as well as with body language. Furniture can be rearranged to avoid eye contact with unwelcome visitors. In an office, the comfort of visitors can be controlled to discourage them from lingering. A closed door can symbolize a management style, preference for isolation, or a need for privacy and confidentiality for specific tasks.

Chairs lined up against the wall in many lounges in institutional settings may facilitate floor maintenance but hinder interpersonal communication. Even if user needs are considered at the time of planning for a new facility, needs change as the population ages or changes. The building and its settings need to be viewed objectively to determine current needs. Has the room changed since the characteristics and abilities of the residents have changed? How has the building changed to meet the new needs of patients/residents who have been there for a long time?

Lounges are generally not very lively places in long-term care facilities. Television is often the center of attention, but residents are usually too far from the set to see it or hear it (although large screens are helpful). Yet the room is arranged for television watching rather than for conversation. If encouragement of socialization is a goal, furniture arrangement that deters side-to-side interaction and eye contact is a problem. Therefore, ganged, in-line seating and long tables should be avoided. The wrong purchase can affect long-term flexibility and options for change. Square tables are often preferred over round tables because they provide more options for space use. They can be paired into a rectangle and provide a clearly defined territorial space for their users.

Territorial behavior prevents residents from sitting next to someone with whom they may want to talk. Sometimes they may be shouting across the room to talk to a friend while still protecting their ownership of the chair and space. Assess whether there is a need to separate smokers and nonsmokers, television watchers and nontelevision watchers. Clear, distinct boundaries can allow separate activities in one room. There is some evidence that when people are provided with well-defined private spaces, they tend to be less withdrawn. Some withdraw without physically leaving the room. It may be the only way to get a degree of privacy in an institutional setting.

Take the time to look around the building with a fresh point of view, looking at the environment as a tool to achieve both organizational and personal goals.

Empathy

Several years ago, while working in a nursing facility, an extended period of observation and a dose of empathy revealed a common environmental problem (Deutschman 1980). A resident entered a multipurpose room in a wheelchair. She asked an aide if it was lunchtime. The aide replied that the woman must have forgotten *again* that she had already eaten lunch and it was nearly dinnertime. A look around the room revealed no sensory cues to trigger her memory and to help her function appropriately. There was no clock in the room, no menu posted to remind her of a meal she had eaten, no smell of food, and no tablecloths on the tables. Trays were wheeled in on carts from another part of the building. She had no environmental clues to tell her it was mealtime. The environment failed to support her needs or encourage her to function independently. At this stage of her life, she is in need of "redundant cueing"—more rather than fewer environmental clues to help her function. Installation of clocks and menu boards were part of the solution. The other missing component was staff awareness that their encouragement through verbal reinforcement serves as a reminder to use these supports.

Observation of a dining room in another nursing facility revealed captain's chairs with arms so short that most of the less competent residents could easily lose their balance when they pulled away from the table; lap trays so high that they reached almost to the resident's armpits making self-feeding very difficult; table heights at a level that made it impossible for patients in wheelchairs to get close enough to the table to eat without dropping food into their laps; table pedestals preventing four residents in wheelchairs from comfortably sharing footroom under the table; and a resident sitting with her feet dangling six to eight inches off the floor because she was propped up in order to reach table height. The standard furniture that was purchased to accommodate a healthier, more independent and mobile population was no longer appropriate. The congestion made mealtime chaotic. Most residents were now being fed by a staff member seated at an adjoining chair. Progressively more people were in wheelchairs partially because it was easier than transferring a person; it was more comfortable; and there was no ambulation program to encourage mobility.

Fortunately, in this facility, members of an environmental committee made up of staff representing all the disciplines, called these problems to the attention of administration. A survey form was distributed to staff and visitors. The cooperation and responses were excellent. The result was an identification of the most frequently mentioned environmental problems. Residents were interviewed and observed.

Was the survey necessary if most of these problems were already noted? The survey helps to give people a sense of empathy and involvement. This information was gathered and analyzed objectively by an outside source. The results should be observable and verifiable without distortion by personal feelings of one or two individuals, as so often occurs when changes are proposed. The survey is part of an education process for all staff and even for visitors. The survey feedback session helps to set priorities. The staff members were assisted to solve their own problems in three separate dining rooms where resident's needs had changed significantly. This facility was ready to purchase furniture, and needed assistance to make the best choices. In addition to space planning and furniture specification, special modular units were designed to accommodate the needs of staff who were feeding residents.

Large numbers of staff were involved in the survey. The environmental committee maintained involvement in setting priorities for the spaces. The facilitators simply helped to clarify issues, to focus on the priorities, and to provide short-term assistance where the committee lacked the expertise to identify their options. With each facility, there are common problems but there is also room for unique solutions. This is an education process that builds staff commitment to making the changes "work." When the time had come to replace the furniture, this input from all levels of staff was valuable to identify such specific needs. Those who spend the time with residents may be most aware of the individual requirements for optimum functioning.

Empathy combined with an objective look at the environment may also help discover upholstered furniture that is too low, too soft, too deep, or too stiff for most residents. The elderly prefer a high back, arms, and padding on chairs, especially for long-duration sitting. Suppliers are very cooperative in providing chairs for evaluation by staff and residents.

Sensitivity

This is the most difficult attribute when addressing environmental issues. Even if staff may already be sensitive to their own needs and to the needs of those in their care, the physical space is usually not a high priority issue with administration or staff. Some professionals perceive it as a frill—simply decoration or ornamentation of wall, floor, or ceiling surfaces—not recognizing environmental sensitivity as a tool to effective, low-cost change in the physical space, thus influencing the behavior of its users.

For example, many facilities have no staff lounge at all. "It's really important to have a comfortable staff lounge, a place to relax, to be away from the job for awhile, a place for staff only," is a comment heard frequently. In one facility, staff members were observed locking the door to a resident activity room, thereby depriving residents of activity space, in order to meet their own needs for privacy and informal meeting space. There is some evidence indicating that if people cannot get away from others when their aggressive impulses are high, they are more likely to act out these impulses. "We need a lounge where you can go on a break without being disturbed by patients and bells," said one staff member. Residents often share space with staff. Many newly designed facilities are no more sensitive to these needs than are the old facilities. Architects still find that administrators expect that their employees will spend too much time in a comfortable lounge.

Lack of privacy is characteristic of health-care settings. Sensitivity to this need reveals that there is a lack of privacy for telephone calls and for family visits in these buildings. There is a special need for privacy for those who share space with a roommate. Privacy is also violated by thoughtless staff. In a survey of six health-care facilities (Deutschman 1982), staff members themselves identified this problem, citing examples of their own peers shouting private facts about residents in public areas such as halls and dining rooms. At the minimum, personal privacy for hygiene and toileting should be respected. In the home environment, if an elderly relative is living with the family, privacy space is equally important for all family members. To determine the appropriate amount of privacy for different people, it is necessary to understand the user's style, needs, and what he or she is trying to do. Residents should have control over the type and the level of interaction. Those who are institutionalized perceive themselves to have significantly less choice than noninstitutionalized individuals. Choice must be built into the physical environment. This includes a variety of spatial settings with choice in visual and other sensory stimuli.

If the health-care facility is large, visitors, residents, and sometimes staff may be seen emerging from the elevator onto the wrong floor, or searching for a specific entrance. Signs may be confusing or difficult to read. Signs at elevators and those identifying rooms and floors may need to be larger, with greater contrast in lightness or darkness from the background color. Visually impaired residents show greater stress because they have greater difficulty seeing interim and ultimate destinations.

Institutionalized elderly persons may need a wide range of auditory and tactile landmarks clearly visible and distinctive. If the facility is relatively new, a coherent, coordinated system of signs was, more than likely, developed when the facility first opened, but if it was never clearly understood and reinforced by staff, a hodge-podge of different signs of different colors, sizes, and placement may exist. An overload of printed information scattered throughout the building can be properly categorized and organized into clearly defined bulletin boards.

A sensitive look at the needs of the elderly in their home, or in an institution, may reveal that they are bored, with nothing to do, especially on weekends, afternoons, and evenings. In the home, discussion followed by a little creativity may suggest options. In a nursing home, recreational materials should not be locked up for the weekend or in the evenings. The key word in milieu therapy is "activity." It's important to reinforce activities of self-care, socialization, desirable behavior, and personal responsibility with increased options for activities suitable for individual needs. Watching the behavior of others is a favorite pastime for residents. In an institution or in housing for the elderly, passive observation of activity areas, rather than hallway traffic, may stimulate participation when residents can see and hear others engaged in activities. Many residents may be escaping from their shared room. Do barriers in resident rooms limit the movement of both staff and residents? Is space in patient bathrooms too limited for independent use? Design of resident rooms should encourage self-maintenance: bathing, dressing, eating, toileting, and walking.

Do all rooms look alike, resulting in confusion for patients? If the same paint color or the same wallcovering is used throughout the building, orientation of residents is not being assisted. Accessibility, adaptability, and normalization should be the objectives in the home and institutional environments.

To summarize, in developing *environmental competence,* the following five-step procedure is recommended:

STEP ONE: Take a fresh new look at your home or institution. Walk through it as you would if you were an outsider making a decision about whether or not you would want to live here or work here.

STEP TWO: Put yourself in the place of residents or staff members. Observe and get a feeling for what it must be like to walk in their shoes, in their personal space. This can't always be done in five minutes. The empathy gained may solve communication problems that are worth the effort and time.

STEP THREE: Force youself to do this not once, but on an ongoing basis, so that objective assessment of the environment becomes part of the process of evaluating a situation in an attempt to solve problems. Manipulation of the environment can become a problem-solving tool. Try it. A low-cost, or no-cost, solution may emerge.

STEP FOUR: When these attempts meet with success, consider an ongoing team effort within work groups or family groups. Satisfaction results from seeing the work group's or the caregivers' effort at change and its favorable influence on the behavior of others. It serves as a positive reinforcement for further improvements.

STEP FIVE: Task forces or committees can effectively deal with specific issues of environmental barriers, input on furniture purchases, and successful coordination of larger changes in the physical space, those requiring the involvement of architects and interior designers. The communication barrier that exists between those who plan and design spaces and those who use them could be effectively reduced. Decisions about the physical environment should be based on specific goals and objectives for the organization and its people rather than on the personal preference of a committee member who is not even a user of the space.

ORGANIZATIONAL CULTURE

If changes in the physical environment are to be used strategically, symbolically, therapeutically, and creatively, it's important to understand and assess the organizational culture typically found in long-term care facilities. Each facility is different but there are some commonalities. It is the staff members who help to identify needs and implement and reinforce change on behalf of residents in long-term care. They exist in a culture that supports or discourages their efforts.

There are two perspectives of organizational culture. One views culture as an organization's system of values, norms, beliefs, and structures that persist over time rather than just at any given moment. Another perspective of organizational culture treats it as both process and context seeking to discover "sense making" devices used by organization members (Weick 1979). Cultural change may be internally induced. Messages can be designed and introduced into an organization's environment to alter its culture (Barnett 1987). However, research indicates that organizations tend to retain old perceptions and patterns of behavior even in the presence of change agents (Falcione & Kaplan 1984). Although rapid, radical change is usually resisted, slow and adaptive change or enrichment may be possible.

Mintzberg (1979) describes a process of "pigeonholing" used by healthcare professionals to facilitate problem solving. Weick (1976) refers to it as "the business of building and maintaining categories." It involves categorizing the client's needs in terms of a contingency, which indicates a standard program to use (diagnosis), and to apply or execute that program. Like stereotypes, these categories allow movement through the job without making continuous decisions (Perrow 1970). Care and units are arranged to help each patient to fit into a category of behavior defined by society. Staff members attempt to change patients' behavior so that it fits their own standards of "normality." The adaptively-structured milieu responds to a more relativistic environmental pressure, so that the very definition of normality is a product of interaction between staff and patients.

In pigeonholing, thought processes are convergent to minimize the possibility of mistakes. Needs that fall at the margin tend to get forced artificially into one category or another. This pigeonholing process can emerge as the source of conflict over continual reassessment of contingencies, imperfectly conceived in programs that are artificially distinguished.

Registered nurses and licensed practical nurses come to their jobs in long-term care with a license confiming their technological skills. Healthcare aides do not. In any case, technological skills do not guarantee attitudes appropriate to the culture. Turnover rates—the proportion of nurses and aides who voluntarily terminate their work in nursing homes in a given period of time—are alarmingly high, reported as high as 240 percent in some facilities. The turnover rate among aides is the highest proportion of the total.

Halbur and Fears (1986) suggest turnover rates of nursing personnel may have positive as well as negative effects, by introducing innovative ideas to nursing homes, easing various changes, and improving standards of care. Turnover may bring in registered nurses who have fresh ideas, thereby enabling the organization to adapt more adequately to internal demands and environmental pressures.

However, average annual turnover rates in nursing facilities range between 55 and 75 percent, exceeding the level of 50 percent that is considered problematic for organizational effectiveness and, perhaps, for survival (Halbur & Fears 1986). Dissatisfaction and burnout are common complaints among staff. Cleek and Karuza (1985) found that burnout results in less time spent with residents. Research reveals that work relationships, social support, and social feedback are modifiers of burnout in many human service organizations (Sypher & Ray 1984; Pines & Kafry 1978).

How organization members make sense of their work environment is largely due to interaction with others in the organization. What may be stressful in one organization may be ignored in another. Ray (1983) suggests that burnout begins when employees are unable to maintain their initial dedication and commitment, and the worker attempts to psychologically distance self from the job. Detachment precedes burnout. Burnout can certainly occur for the caregiver at home as well.

Most job turnover studies indicate the first few months of a new employee's tenure are critical in the development of healthy attitudes and behavior patterns. This period is likely to include significant ambiguity, stress, and anxiety.

From an organizational communication perspective, after the first few days on the job, newcomers begin to move from the anticipation stage to the stage of testing and revising expectations. This is accompanied by attempts at "sense-making," questioning, assessing opportunities and constraints. New employees move into an existing set of formal and informal relationships. They are expected to behave in ways that support and perpetuate the culture (Conrad 1985). Through social activities, new members learn meanings of symbols and the attitudes, values, and beliefs common to members. Culture is communicated through an organization's informal interpersonal networks (Rogers & Agarwala-Rogers 1976). Deviance from shared standards is not tolerated. For example, in New York State, nursing homes are now required to provide 100 hours of training for the health-care aides. After their training, the "old guard" assures adherence to the existing norms where the training deviates from those norms.

This encounter stage for a newcomer involves learning the culture, assessing behavioral expectations, and developing task-related skills. The first step in developing long-term skills is a need to determine career paths. Health-care aides soon discover there are no career paths for them in this setting. This is one of the reasons for the high turnover rates among aides.

Jablin (1984) reported on a longitudinal, developmental study of the process by which new employees, nursing assistants (aides) in nursing homes, are assimilated into their organization's communication systems. Time was a major independent variable affecting development of organizational communication attitudes and behaviors. This continuous process can be divided into two parts: (1) the organization's efforts to socialize the new employee, which occurs in sequential phases of reconstruction of him/her, and (2) the new employee's attempts to individualize his or her role in the organization. Here the superior is of central importance in the employee's favorable or unfavorable perceptions of the organization.

Role stress results from lack of, or distortion of, downward communication from the supervisor (Fulk & Mani 1986). Jablin (1984) suggests that if a new employee's immediate supervisor understands a recruit's "sensemaking" of the organization, this increases the probability of the new employee's effective assimilation into the organization.

Jablin found that *lower* expectations on the part of the new recruit resulted in *increased* likelihood of job survival. Most new employees tend to focus on superiors for the purpose of receiving information to learn behavioral and attitudinal norms. They tend to wait for others to supply them with relevant information in the early stages of employment. Their interactions with patients are for the purpose of giving information and were reported to be significantly less positive than attitudes toward interactions with peers and superiors. Jablin found that health-care supervisors tend to communicate expectations of recruit *dissatisfaction* with their jobs and with their employers.

In long-term care settings, where aide-level staff members have the most contact with residents, their access to psychosocial information regarding the residents may be very valuable in decison making and environmental change. Use of this input requires organizational norms that permit influence to be based on knowledge and information rather than on hierarchical position. In most long-term care facilities, a culture change and changes in communication regularities are required to create these norms. How can the norms change if nonconformity to existing norms is frowned upon and is seen as behavior that serves selfish motives?

There are good reasons for changing norms. Without supportive norms, if the strategies of the subordinate succeed, sometimes they threaten the superiority, self-esteem, and self-image of power holders. Powerful people can refuse to use participatory strategies, use them only for trivial issues, split the group, impede its ability to make effective decisions, withhold valuable information, sabotage the decision, or refuse to carry out the decision (Conrad 1985).

Supervisors tend to have more education and greater communication skills than subordinates. They are often more persuasive, argue positions more effectively, and are more adept at interpreting and responding to communication. These advantages allow them to influence views of other members of a group. People with high levels of communication anxiety may find participation to be very threatening with their superiors present, and may respond by withdrawing from the discussion. When employees have either less opportunity to participate than they desire or more than they wish, stress and lower quality of performance may result (Conrad 1985). Findings generally imply that the more open, trusting, and participative the superior-subordinate relationship is perceived to be by the subordinate, the more satisfied the subordinate is likely to be with the job or with the organization (Richmond, Wagner & McCroskey 1981).

In a recent study by Deutschman (1988), an across-shift and across-level communication strategy was devised to enable staff members to collaborate on the introduction of strategic change in the personal space/territory of residents in a long-term care facility. Staff were very cooperative until the time of implementation and reinforcement. There was very little reinforcement of interventions. Comments given verbally included "morale is so low," "excellent care but poor attitude," "more work piled on," "more paper work," "too many house-cleaning duties for aides, less time for patients," "aides get dumped on," "no time for creativity." Yet the shared information from each shift on each resident was read with great interest by staff. In a retrospective questionnaire, 76 percent of the responding staff wanted some cross-shift communication process to be developed. They submitted a mean of 4.5 creative recommendations per resident to the project, so their creativity is evidence that they are not apathetic or pessimistic.

Kahana and Kiyak (1985) found that the more staff worked with residents, the more negative stereotypes were reinforced. They reported more negative stereotyping occurred among the day shift, among the less educated staff, the younger staff, and among the lower status jobs, such as aides. Solomon (1983) suggests, "Health care providers perceive the long-term outcome to be negative and the costs in terms of emotional and physical energy to be high. Therefore, they are unlikely to invest much energy to minimize cost and maximize the few benefits to be gained from working with the elderly. Their behavior becomes responsive to their own needs to optimize their own 'cost/benefit ratio,' and may become unresponsive to the elderly patient. Thus, response-outcome becomes independent of the elderly patient's response to stimuli."

Solomon further suggests that "the health care provider who treats the elderly patient in a way inconsistent with stereotyping, and who perceives working with the elderly as having long-term benefits at lesser costs than perceived by colleagues, can expect to meet with the disapproval of colleagues." So the system of stereotyping is maintained and the elderly "play the game" by the provider's rules, accepting passivity and dependency.

Unless the rules of the game are changed, the long-term health-care system will maintain high turnover and absenteeism and unbalanced interpersonal relationships. "The way we do things around here" is communicated by observable behaviors. This, in turn, produces norms that shape behaviors by pressure to conform or by ostracism.

Since there is no strong evidence that health-care aides have a desire for challenging and meaningful work, a learning theory, rather than a motivation theory, may be appropriate to effect change in both aide and resident behaviors. Behavior may actually be shaped into what is desired. Shaping is a particularly important technique in behavior modification if a desired response is not currently in a person's behavior repertoire (Luthans & Kreitner 1975). Modeling techniques may be effective with staff using in-person demonstrations and/or training films, slides, or video. Progress of the modeled behavior is praised. Effective supervisor-subordinate inter-actions would focus on a few learning points.

The process of shaping can be very effective with those residents whose deficiencies limit their independent functioning. Baltes and Wahl (1985) have focused on the influence of the social environmental conditions on dependent and independent behaviors of the elderly. It is recommended here that the physical environment could be used as a tool in these interactive sequences of observable staff-resident behavior.

Are dependent behaviors in the elderly reversible or capable of modi-fication using these techniques? Baltes (1982) found change procedures con-sisting of stimulus, control, and reinforcement were most effective with a seventy-nine-year-old man whose overall dependency was due, in large part, to the effects of a stroke. Providing the man with more adequate eating utensils, and then providing immediate social praise following any act of self-feeding, was most effective. The combination of prosthetic environmental intervention and therapeutic reinforcement were most successful in changing behavior.

Training of the aide, which must be supervised by nurses, could include formal techniques of shaping appropriate behavior and using environmental competence as a tool. Nurses who have been communicating an expectation of job dissatisfaction to aides, could expect shaping to pay off in more independent behavior in residents, as a result of aide efforts. Both these relationships could be influenced in a positive direction. The resident who has been rewarded for dependent behavior would now be rewarded for independent, skill-building learning behavior, which would be reinforced because of the rewards gained by the aide in his/her role.

An array of aids and devices used by occupational therapists for the elderly in the community could be made available for appropriate use by health-care aides for behavior modification exchanges with residents. Helping relationships need to be tailored to each specific person-environment combination rather than applied uniformly to elderly nursing home residents. Staff members need to take into account tremendous differences between elderly individuals.

Most of the behaviors of the elderly are expressed in the form of compliance or cooperation. Most of the behaviors of staff and family take the form of a request/command/suggestion or cooperation. Boredom in the setting increases the high frequency of withdrawal behaviors. In a number of situations, the elderly are able to perform the required behavior but they are prevented from doing so by the immediate help from staff. Baltes suggests that the *one* behavior that has the highest probability of securing supportive or attentive behavior from staff or family is *dependent* self-care behavior. This is one sure way to have social contact. Staff training can change behavior from dependent-supportive to independent-supportive but some dependence should be accepted as an expression of successful aging, states Baltes. Dependency may represent a way to experience passive control in a highly constraining environment (Baltes & Reisenzein 1985).

Staff training in basic skills and attitudes should include addressing the resident as he or she prefers; always telling the resident what procedure is to be performed, how long it will take or what to expect; learning the resident's likes and dislikes, what the resident perceives as his/her greatest problems, what expectations the resident has about the nursing home; permitting the resident to keep up with hobbies and avocations. Nurses ought to know at least as much about residents as the nursing assistants (Goodwin & Trocchio 1987).

In the commercial world, if products are not right on target, people will find products that are. Every employee of Worthington, a steel processor based in Columbus, Ohio, carries the company's "golden rule" on a card stating "we treat customers, employees, investors, and suppliers as we would like to be treated." Corporate America's sudden interest in listening to customers marks a big departure (Glaberson 1988). When will long-term health care begin listening to its various constituencies?

THE ELDERLY IN THE PUBLIC ENVIRONMENT

One of the areas thus far ignored in this chapter is the public spaces— the public buildings, public transportation, parks, and other community environments. It's important to remember that aging is as individual as one's fingerprint. Most elderly people are perfectly able to carry on normal activities. Being elderly, healthy, and active in the community may be no different from being middle-aged, healthy, and active. Being elderly with a disability may be no different from being middle-aged with a disability.

Unfortunately, environments are constructed to facilitate the activities of able-bodied people.

Some existing environments have been modified to allow people with disabilities to use them competently. Accesibility and adaptability are key issues for those who have a handicapping condition. To assist with mobility problems, it's important to create awareness of hazardous objects in or near their path of travel; to provide aids and information helpful in finding one's way and in orientation; to use tactile or auditory signals for the visually impaired to warn of upcoming hazards.

Older people of both sexes tend to be shorter than younger people. Reach measurements of older people are shorter than those of their younger counterparts. If reach is a critical factor in the design of a public space, it is essential to base the design not on the average, but on the lower range of the population in order to accommodate more than 50 percent of that population. There is also considerable variability in the elderly due to the incidence of arthritis and other joint movement limitation.

It's important to view the chairbound person as an individual together with the wheelchair. This requires some observation of the anatomy of the wheelchair itself. Most wheelchairs are not built to keep the body in an erect position. The average turning space for a wheelchair is five feet. Provision of ramps and other assistance for those functioning with a disability in public buildings has assisted the elderly as well.

For the ambulatory disabled, it is necessary to consider those functioning with crutches, walkers, and canes. Changes of grade and circulation up and down stairs are extremely difficult or may be impossible in some situations for those with crutches. Limited use of extremities as well as manipulation and placement of crutches significantly limits leverage, especially when opening or closing doors or getting in and out of seats. A walker requires a minimum of twenty-eight inches (Panero & Zelnik 1979).

A clear separation between vehicular traffic and pedestrian traffic should be assured. Gradients should be gentle with provision of good runoff of surface water to minimize standing water that will freeze in cold weather. Public seating should be available at intervals to permit resting.

Location of housing for the elderly should be in an active community context. Care should be taken to ensure that public transportation is available for residents and visitors to permit a high level of interaction between the elderly and the community. Residents should continue to participate in local community and family activities including churches, clubs, shopping, and visits from friends and relatives. Volunteers are important in the success of facilities for the elderly.

Areas protected from both the sun and wind should be created outdoors for casual sitting. These areas should offer views of both community activity and the main entrance. Judicious use of fences, screens, and planting should ensure protection of outdoor areas from unwanted intrusion (Cluff 1979). Privacy and security are top priorities, but, at the same time, it is important to provide opportunities for the elderly to observe activity. The provision of adequate lighting is important for security and mobility. Handrails and supports should be provided along pathways and stairs. Irregular walking surfaces, whether hazardous or only perceived as hazardous, will influence mobility. High curbs can also restrict mobility.

SUMMARY

The environment communicates to those who use it, transmitting messages about appropriate behavior and meanings. If the environment, that area outside the skin, can be modified to meet the needs of elderly persons and their caregivers, then in effect, their competence has increased because they are provided with help to adapt to their circumstances. For those who interact with the elderly, the development of objectivity, empathy, and sensitivity are important steps in learning how the users experience the environment. Before change can take place, analysis and observation is required to convey some sense of how the aged feel as their options become limited due to sensory impairment, social isolation, and, for some, institutionalization. How are individual residents coping? What is the culture in which they and their caregivers exist? What training is required? Does the system support and encourage innovation? Some of the stereotypic views of our society are carried into the health-care setting by those who enter, including staff members. Communication is a key factor in the process by which the resident sizes up and adapts to a new situation. Family members with awareness, and well-trained staff, can help in the adaptation and adjustment process. Appropriate environments offer the elderly individual dignity, privacy, and independence combined with a sense of self-worth and purpose.

FOR DISCUSSION

1. What theories would lead you to believe that changes in the physical environment can influence the quality of life for the elderly?
2. What effect does staff burnout have on the environment for the elderly and on the culture of a long-term facility?
3. List at least twenty changes in the physical space of the home of sensory impaired elderly persons that would permit them to continue to live safely and independently.

116   Working with the Elderly

4. Compile a list of sensory changes and nonverbal factors that influence the life of the elderly.
5. Describe the specific steps one could use to achieve the objectivity, empathy, and sensitivity required for the development of environmental competence.

REFERENCES

Aging America. "Trends and Projections." Prepared by the U.S. Senate Committee on Aging, in conjunction with the American Association of Retired Persons, the Federal Council on the Aging, and the Administration on Aging. 1985-1986 edition.

Baltes, M. M. "Dependency in the Elderly." Paper presented at the 38th annual scientific meeting of the Gerontological Society of America, New Orleans, November 1985.

———. "Environmental Factors in Dependency among Nursing Home Residents: A Social Ecology Analysis." In T. A. Wills (ed.) *Basic Processes in Helping Relationships.* New York: Academic Press, 1982, pp. 405-425.

Baltes, M. M., and Reisenzein, R. "The Social World in Long-Term Care Institutions: Psychological Control Toward Dependency?" In M. M. Baltes and P. B. Baltes (eds.) *The Psychology of Control and Aging.* Hillsdale, N.J.: Erlbaum, 1985.

Baltes, M. M. and Wahl, H. W. "Dependency in Aging." In L. L. Cartensen and B. Y. Edelstein (eds.) *Handbook of Clinical Gerontology.* New York: Pergamon Press, 1985.

Barnett, G. A. "Communication and Organizational Culture." In G. M. Goldhaber (ed.) *Handbook of Organizational Communication.* Norwood, N.J.: Ablex Publishing Co., 1987.

Brink, T. L. *Geriatric Psychotherapy.* New York: Human Sciences Press. 1979.

Burgoon, J. K. "Privacy and Communication." In M. Burgoon (ed.) *Communication Yearbook 6.* Beverly Hills, Calif.: Sage Publications, 1982, pp. 206-249.

Cleek, M. A., and Karuza, J. "Institutional Staff's Impact on Quality and Cost of Care: A Needed Focus." A symposium presented at the 38th annual scientific meeting of the Gerontological Society of America, New Orleans, November 1985.

Cluff, P. *Nursing Homes and Hostels with Care Services for the Elderly: Design Guidelines.* Canada Mortgage and Housing Corporation, 1979.

Conrad, C. *Strategic Organizational Communication: Cultures, Situations, and Adaptation.* New York: Holt, Rinehart and Winston, 1985.

Cooper, B., Gowland, C., and McIntosh, J. "The Use of Color in the Environment of the Elderly to Enhance Function." *Clinical Geriatric Medicine* 2, no. 1, February (1986): 151-163.

Deal, T. E., and Kennedy, A. A. *Corporate Cultures: The Rites and Rituals of Corporate Life*. Reading, Mass.: Addison-Wesley, 1982.

Deutschman, M. "A Communication Process for Environmental Management to Affect Changes in Functional Levels of Residents in a Long-Term Care Facility." Ph.D dissertation, State University of New York at Buffalo, 1988.

————. "Environmental Competence and Environmental Management." *The Journal of Long-Term Care Administration,* Fall (1985): 78-84.

————. "Environmental Settings and Environmental Competence." *Gerontology and Geriatrics Education* 2, no. 3, (Spring 1982): 237-242.

————. "Environment and Productivity." *Contemporary Administrator* (January 1980): 10-14.

————. "How Can You Get Your Building to Work?" *American Health Care Association Journal* (January 1980): 20-22.

Falcione, R. L., and Kaplan, E. A. "Organizational Climate, Communication, and Culture." In R. Bostrom (ed.) *Communication Yearbook 8*. Beverly Hills, Calif.: Sage Publications, 1984.

Fulk, J., and Mani, S. "Distortion in Hierarchical Relationships." In M. McLaughlin (ed.) *Communication Yearbook 9*. Beverly Hills, Calif.: Sage Publications, 1986, pp. 483-510.

Glaberson, W. "Listening to the Consumer Again." *The New York Times* (April 6, 1988).

Goldhaber, G. M. *Organizational Communication*. Dubuque, Iowa: Wm. C. Brown Co., 1983.

Goodwin, M., and Trocchio, J. "Cultivating Positive Attitudes in Nursing Home Staff." *Geriatric Nursing* (January/February 1987).

Greenberg, C. I., and Firestone, I. J. "Compensatory Responses to Crowding: Effects of Personal Space Intrusion and Privacy Reduction." *Journal of Personality and Social Psychology* 35 (1977): 637-644.

Greene, J. A. "Management Techniques Unique in Special Alzheimer Unit." *Provider* (September 1986): 41-42.

Halbur, B. T. and Fears, N. "Nursing Personnel Turnover Rates Turned Over: Potential Positive Side Effects on Resident Outcomes in Nursing Homes." *The Gerontologist* 26, no. 1 (February 1986): 70-76.

Hall, E. T. *The Silent Language*. Garden City, N.Y.: Anchor Books, 1973.

Harel, Z. "Quality of Care, Congruence and Well-Being among Institutionalized Aged." *The Gerontologist* 21, no. 5 (October 1981): 523-531.

Hiatt, L. "The Environment as a Participant in Health Care." *Journal of Long Term Care Administration* 10, no. 2 (1982): 2-7.

Jablin, F. M. "Assimilating New Members into Organizations." In R. Bostrom (ed.) *Communication Yearbook 8.* Beverly Hills, Calif.: Sage Publications, 1984, pp. 594-626.

Kahana, E. A. "Confrontations with Diverse Stresses in Late Life." Presentation at the Western New York Geriatric Center 1988 Faculty Development Program, March 30, 1988.

Kahana, E. A., and Kiyak, H. A. "Personal and Job Related Predictors of Employee Turnover in Facilities for the Elderly." Paper presented at symposium—M. Cleek and J. Karuza (Chairs), at the 38th Annual Scientific Meeting of the Gerontological Society of America. New Orleans, November 1985.

Kahana, L., Liang, J., and Felton, B. "Alternative Models of Person-Environment Fit: Prediction of Morale in Three Homes for the Aged." *Journal of Gerontology* 35 (July 1980): 584-595.

Kayser-Jones, J. S. "Open-Ward Accommodations in a Long-Term Care Facility: The Elderly's Point of View." *The Gerontologist* 26, 1 (February 1986): 63-69.

———. "The Prevention of Falls in Later Life." A report by the Kellogg International Work Group on the Prevention of Falls by the Elderly (April 1987).

Langer, E. J. "The Illusion of Control." *Journal of Personality and Social Psychology* 32 (1975).

Lawton, M. P. "Environment and the Well-Being of Older People." Presentation at the Western New York Geriatric Center 1988 Faculty Development Program (March 16, 1988).

———. "Competence, Environmental Press and the Adaptation of Older People." In P. Windley, T. Byerts, and F. Ernst (eds.) *Theory Development in Environment and Aging.* Washington, D.C.: Gerontological Society, 1975, pp. 13-84.

———. "Ecology and Aging." In L. D. Pastalan and D. H. Carson (eds.) *Spatial Behavior of Older People.* Ann Arbor, Mich.: University of Michigan Press, 1970.

Lawton, M. P., and Nahemow, L. "Ecology and the Aging Process." In C. Eisdorfer and M. P. Lawton (eds.) *The Psychology of Adult Development and Aging.* Washington, D.C.: American Psychological Association, 1973.

Lawton, M. P., and Simon, B. B. "The Ecology of Social Relationships in Housing for the Elderly." *The Gerontologist* 8 (1968): 108-115.

Luthans, F., and Kreitner, R. "The Role of Punishment in Organizational Behavior Modification." *Public Personnel Management* 2, no. 3, 156-161.

Mintzberg, H. *The Structuring of Organizations.* Englewood Cliffs, N.J.: Prentice-Hall Inc., 1979.

Nehrke, M. F., Morganti, J. B., Cohen, S. H., Hulicka, I. M., Whitbourne, S. K., Turner, R. R., and Cataldo, J. F. "Differences in Person-Environment Congruence Between Micro-Environments." *Canadian Journal on Aging* 3 (1984): 117-132.

Nehrke, M. F., Whitbourne, S. K., Cataldo, J. F., Cohen, S. H., Turner, R. R., Morganti, J. B. and Hulicka, I. M. "P-E Congruence Prediction of Well-Being: A Longitudinal Study." Presented at the 36th annual meeting of the Gerontological Society of America, San Francisco, 1983.

Nehrke, M. F., Turner, R. R., Cohen, S. H., Whitbourne, S. K., Morganti, J. B., and Hulicka, I. M. "Toward a Model of Person-Environment Congruence: Development of the EPPIS." *Experimental Aging Research* 7 (1981): 363-380.

Nelson, F. L., and Farberow, N. L. "Indirect Self-Destructive Behavior in the Elderly Nursing Home Patient." *Journal of Gerontology* 35, no. 6 (1980): 949-957.

Nicholson, C. K., and Nicholson, J. I. *The Personalized Care Model for the Elderly.* Chittenango, N.Y.: Nicholson & Nicholson. 1982.

Panero, J., and Zelnik, M. *Human Dimension and Interior Space.* New York: Watson-Guptill Publications, 1979.

Pastalan, L. D. "Environmental Graphics Design Conference." Cranbrook Academy, Michigan, 1980.

Patterson, A. H. "Territorial Behavior and Fear of Crime in the Elderly." *Environmental Psychology and Nonverbal Behavior* 2 (1978): 131-144.

Perrow, C. *Organizational Analysis: A Sociological Review.* Belmont, Calif.: Wadsworth, 1970.

Pines, A., and Kafry, D. "Occupational Tedium in Social Services." *Social Work* (November 1978): 499-507.

Proch, V. "Promoting Meaningful Long-Term Care Experiences: One Dean's View." In *Creating a Choice for Nurses: Long-Term Care.* New York: National League for Nursing (publication no. 20-1917), 1983.

Ray, E. B. "Job Burnout from a Communication Perspective." In R. N. Bostrom (ed.) *Communication Yearbook 7.* Beverly Hills, Calif.: Sage Publications, 1983, pp. 738-755.

Richmond, V. P., Wagner, J. P., and McCroskey, J. C. "The Impact of Perceptions of Leadership Style, Use of Power, and Conflict Management Style on Organizational Outcomes." *Communication Quarterly* 31 (1981): 27-36.

Rogers, E. M., and Rogers, R. A. *Communication in Organizations.* New York: The Free Press. 1976.

Rosenthal, R. *Skill in Nonverbal Communication: Individual Differences.* Cambridge, Mass.: Oelgeschlager, Bunn and Hain, 1979.

Ryden, M. "Environmental Support for Autonomy in the Institutionalized Elderly." *Research in Nurse Health* 8, no. 4 (December 1985): 363-371.

Solomon, K. "Victimization by Health Professionals and the Psychologic Response of the Elderly." In J. I. Kosberg (ed.) *The Abuse and Maltreatment of the Elderly.* Littleton: John Wright—PSG Publishing, 1983, pp. 150-171.

Steele, F. I. *Physical Settings and Organizational Behavior.* Reading, Mass.: Addison-Wesley, 1973.

Stein, S., Linn, M. W., and Stein, E. M. "Patients' Perceptions of Nursing Home Stress Related to Quality of Care." *The Gerontologist* 26, no. 4 (August 1986): 424-430.

Steinfeld, E. "Access to the Built Environment: A Review of the Literature." U.S. Dept. of Housing and Urban Development. Washington, D.C. U.S. Government Printing Office, April 1979.

Stern, G. G. *People in Context.* New York: Wiley, 1970.

Strauss, H., Aldrich, B., and Lipman, A. "Retirement and Perceived Status Loss: An Inquiring into Some Objective and Subjective Problems Produced by Aging." In J. Gubrium (ed.) *Time Roles and Self in Old Age.* New York: Human Sciences. 1976.

Sundstrom, E. "An Experimental Study of Crowding: Effects of Room Size, Intrusion, and Goal Blocking on Nonverbal Behavior, and Self-Reported Stress." *Journal of Personality and Social Psychology* 32 (1975): 645-659.

Sypher, B. D., and Ray, E. B. "Communication and Job Stress in a Health Organization." In R. Bostrom (ed.) *Communication Yearbook 8.* Beverly Hills, Calif.: Sage Publications. 1984.

Thayer, S. "Close Encounters." *Psychology Today* (March 1988): 31-36.

Tobin, S. S., and Lieberman, M. A. *Last Home for the Aged.* San Francisco: Jossey Bass. 1976.

Weick, K. E. *The Social Psychology of Organizing.* Reading, Mass.: Addison-Wesley. 1979.

———. "Educational Organizations as Loosely Coupled Systems." *Administrative Science Quarterly* (1976): 1-19.

Westin, A. *Privacy and Freedom.* New York: Atheneum, 1967.

Zimring, C. M. "Stress and the Designed Environment." *The Journal of Social Issues* 37 (1981): 145-71.

6

The Concept of Service

Rosemary McCaslin

HUMAN SERVICES FOR THE ELDERLY

The term "human services" encompasses a wide range of formal programs and professions that attempt to alleviate suffering and maximize individuals' abilities to participate fully in their community. These services may include, for example, medical care, preventive and rehabilitative health efforts, financial assistance, various forms of counseling, and assistance with necessary daily activities such as cooking and bathing. Specific services may be funded by federal, state, or local government or by private charities. The same type of service may be provided in slightly different ways in various communities to best address local needs.

As people age, they often experience a variety of changes and losses that can constrain their ability to function as independent adults; human services may be needed to offset these changes. Retirement often reduces income, and inflation can further reduce adequacy of what remains. Both normal aging and later-life diseases can make it difficult to manage yard work, household chores, and even personal care. Retirement, poor health, and other changes can result in isolation and few chances to socialize with peers or to contribute to the community. Services exist that can help the elderly with these and many other problems.

It can be difficult to think systematically about the many different human services that might be needed by elderly persons. Particular human services for older persons can be defined as supports for specific deficits in normal adult functioning (Golant & McCaslin 1979). Functional deficits can occur in four broad areas, and services that address each of these will need to be available.

First, all individuals must maintain some degree of health to carry out any other tasks of living. Persons with disabilities, for example, often use special devices (e.g., canes, wheelchairs, and even computers) that minimize the impact of their health problem and allow them to function much as persons who do not have that disability.

Second, all adults must be able to solve problems that arise in day-to-day living, whether these be crises, emotional distresses, or daily hassles. Education is made available to all children and adolescents, in part to prepare them to be adult problem solvers. Since life always brings unexpected events, various professional counselors are needed to help individuals manage the trying times in their lives.

Third, adults are expected to take responsibility for a multitude of tasks that are necessary to maintain themselves as independent members of their community. These tasks include both personal care (e.g., bathing, grooming, wearing appropriate clothes) and meeting the expectations of the outside world (e.g., cleaning house, cutting the grass, paying bills). Health problems encountered in late life often make such tasks difficult and can jeopardize the ability of older persons to remain in their own homes.

Finally, adults must maintain connections with other persons such as family, friends, and neighbors. Social contacts can shrink in late life: family members move, friends die, health and financial problems limit outside activities.

Each of these four areas covers a wide range of potential functions and constraints of an elderly person's abilities. Physical health concerns, for example, range from treatment for serious illness to maintenance of optimal wellness. Since different degrees of impairment can require quite different supports, human services for the elderly must also he made available for persons at different levels of independence. Three broad levels of independence can be used to define needed services: the comparatively well-elderly, elderly needing assistance to prevent premature institutionalization, and the institutionalized or otherwise totally dependent elderly.

When the four areas of adult functioning and three levels of independence are combined, we can consider twelve general categories of human services that may be needed by older persons. An ideal service system would provide some services in each category. Table 1 lists some programs for the elderly that are common today according to these categories. It is easy to see which needs of older people have been given the most attention by human service providers: many programs have been developed, for example, to assist with tasks of daily living and help the elderly stay in their own homes as long as possible. Conversely, it is obvious that human service providers have not yet given much thought to the social needs of those elderly who reside in institutions such as nursing homes.

TABLE 1

HUMAN SERVICE PROGRAMS FOR THE ELDERLY WHICH ARE AVAILABLE IN MANY COMMUNITIES

LEVELS OF INDEPENDENCE

	Health	Problem Solving	Daily Activities	Social Contact
Comparatively Well	Exercise Health clinics Dental clinics	Information & referral Retirement planning Adult education	Legal aid Reduced prices for seniors Employment services	Senior centers Recreation Group travel
Help Needed to Prevent Institutionalization	Home-delivered meals Visiting nurses Food stamps	Individual counseling Family counseling	Homemakers Home repairs Congregate meals	Transportation Friendly visitors
Totally Dependent	Hospitals Nursing homes Hospice	Psychiatric hospitals Day care	Guardianship	Activities program

AREAS OF FUNCTIONING

The particular services available in a given community will vary. By thinking about human services in terms of the functional deficits they support, we can more easily identify gaps in the service system. Additionally, it is possible to consider other services that might meet a particular need better then existing programs. For example, many persons who are now elderly are reluctant to use professional counseling services. Perhaps peer support groups at senior centers would better meet their needs for help in solving problems that occur in late life.

PSYCHOLOGY OF A PERSON ENTERING HUMAN SERVICES

Many types of providers are involved in services to the elderly: doctors, nurses, social workers, art and music therapists, and home health aides, to name a few. These human service providers differ in their years of schooling, degrees earned, areas of specialized knowledge, and ways of thinking about problems encountered in late life. However, they all share at least two things: a desire to help older persons live out their later years with as much comfort and dignity as possible and some special training to turn that desire to help into effective actions.

Human service providers in the field of aging are often asked by outsiders how they keep from being depressed by working with people who are sick, frail, and nearing the end of their lives. Most who work in the field of geriatrics say that, on the contrary, they find the work very rewarding. Many mention how much they learn from their elderly clients in areas ranging from historical facts to the capacity of people to endure hardship and even learn from adversity. This attitude should not be surprising since professionals who choose to work with the elderly are people who like and value the aged. They are also people who derive personal satisfaction from the process of helping other people on an individual basis. Not uncommonly, their own past experiences have had an influence on their choice of careers. They may remember a human service provider who made a difference in their own life and thereby seek to return what they were given through service to others. Or they may have felt very close to an elderly family member and seek to continue the warmth of that relationship in their professional role.

Any career decision should be based, in part, on consideration of whether the work will be satisfying. Yet, paradoxically, the frequently personal motivations of human service providers and the interpersonal nature of their work make it important that training go beyond learning skills to include self-examination. Not every client will benefit from the type of help we ourselves may have received in the past, and not every older person will be like our favorite aunt. The insights we gather in our own lives are very useful but we must also be prepared to help people who are quite unlike ourselves and people we have known.

It has been suggested that human service providers should learn to anticipate similarities and differences between themselves and a given client even before the first meeting (Germain & Gitterman 1980). A four-step process can be used to make the most of their experiences and, at the same time, achieve the objectivity necessary to appreciate each person's uniqueness.

A provider who is about to meet a new client for the first time usually has some minimal information about that person; perhaps, age, gender, and the reason for their visit. Whatever information is available can be considered from multiple perspectives.

Consider the following example. A nurse is about to call on Ms. G., a seventy-five-year-old widow who is making her first visit to a senior health clinic. The referral form indicates that Ms. G. is seeking advice and assistance about severe arthritis in her knees.

First, the nurse attempts to *identify* with Ms. G. by trying to experience what the other person may be thinking and feeling. Recalling what is known about the process of aging, the nurse remembers that arthritis can become progressively severe in late life and that such inflammation in the joints of the knee can make many daily tasks painful if not impossible: walking, bending to pick up a dropped object, and even sitting down or rising from a chair or the toilet. The nurse wonders whether Ms. G. must negotiate any stairs to leave her house and whether she has any family or friends nearby to assist her or to run errands. The nurse also considers what emotions may be connected with a chronic physical problem. Ms. G., the nurse imagines, may be frustrated over her increasing inability to manage her daily affairs. She might also be depressed if she has become homebound and isolated, angry if her children have not been able to help as much as she would like, or frightened if she associates this particular health problem with the stereotype of aging as terminal decline and dependency.

After thinking through as many possible problems and emotions as possible, the nurse attempts to *incorporate* Ms. G.'s situation by feeling the new client's experiences as if they were her own. That is, the nurse goes beyond the safety of only thinking about the client's potential concerns; for a few moments, she lets herself remember how it actually feels to be depressed and afraid.

Next, the nurse lets herself go one step further to let the client's situation *reverberate* with experiences in her own life. Few human service providers who work with the elderly have been old themselves. However, human emotions are universal and occur at all ages. Perhaps the nurse once broke her leg and remembers the frustration and demoralization of months when normal activities were difficult or when she required help from others.

Evoking one's own past experiences not only increases empathy for the client's situation, but also allows the provider to check for personal reactions that might get in the way of helping the client. For example, the nurse's broken leg might have occurred just as she was finishing her training and preparing to establish herself as an independent adult. If, instead, she lived with her parents for an additional six months while the leg healed, she may have experienced larger frustrations over delayed adulthood. In turn, she might have avoided being angry at herself by becoming (irrationally) angry at her parents. It would be important for the nurse to remember such personal elements of her past so they do not color her view of Ms. G.'s unique situation.

Having allowed her own past feelings to surface, the nurse must now remind herself that Ms. G. is a separate person; two people may experience similar feelings but they can never fully know how the other experiences life. As a final step, then, the provider must once again achieve a degree of *detachment,* returning to rational, objective analysis of the client's problems and concerns. The nurse now readies herself to listen to Ms. G. and let the client describe her actual situation. In addition, however, the nurse is now better prepared to understand and appreciate whatever problems and feelings are expressed by Ms. G.

Human service providers must also learn to be sensitive to the difficulty of asking for help from a stranger. This issue is so common among older persons that it deserves further exploration.

BECOMING A CLIENT

Older persons encounter many difficulties that can be eased or alleviated by professionals: illnesses, functional declines, economic problems, family conflicts, and fears of aging and dying. Given the many services that can be of use in late life, we often hear public debate over the potential costs of supporting a growing elderly population. Ironically, actual use of existing community services by older persons is low compared to estimates of need. For example, 15 to 30 percent of elderly persons are estimated to have diagnosable psychiatric symptoms (Finkel et al. 1981; Pfeiffer 1977; Shanas & Maddox 1976), yet only 2 to 4 percent of clients seen in mental health clinics are over the age of sixty-five (Kaplan 1979; Kramer, Taube & Redick 1973; Zarit 1980).

Why some older persons make use of formal services while other, equally needy elders do not, has not been clarified (Krout 1983; McCaslin 1989). Programs such as senior centers and health education that exist to keep the well-elderly fit and active have the highest rates of usage, ranging from 15 to 30 percent among different services and communities. Those elderly who do take advantage of such programs usually attend more than one (McCaslin 1988). For example, a person who goes to the local senior center is also likely to take exercise classes and go on trips organized for seniors at special prices. One the other hand, the large majority of persons over sixty-five take advantage of none of these programs.

Most services that address needs of frail and ill elderly are used by no more than 3 to 5 percent of the population over age sixty-five. Yet, about 16 percent of persons in that age group experience major limitations in daily functioning (Busse 1980). Research has shown that frail elderly persons who need assistance with day-to-day functioning tend to use only one service at a time (McCaslin 1988). For example, an individual might receive home-delivered meals but not have the services of a homemaker, even though health problems that would make it difficult to cook also make it difficult to wash dishes and clean house. Other studies have shown that some elderly overstate their difficulties when asking for help (McCaslin & Calvert 1975), raising the possibility that they feel it is not appropriate to ask for help unless their circumstances are especially severe. One wonders if some frail elderly who need considerable assistance can only bring themselves to request help with the one problem they see as most pressing.

To understand why some people take advantage of available programs while others do not, it is necessary to consider the personal process that must begin even before an individual contacts human service professionals. This process consists of achieving a balance between often competing forces: anxiety, hope, and fear.

ANXIETY AND HOPE: THE PULL TOWARD ASSISTANCE

People come to human service providers for help with some problem that causes them concern or discomfort and that they are not able to solve on their own. They may lack the skills or knowledge necessary to solve the problem; when an illness does not respond to home remedies, they seek the advice of a health-care professional. These individuals may encounter a problem that is new to them; the restricted income of retirement may require different techniques of financial management than those that were used to manage monthly income from employment.

Concern about a problem and inability to solve it on one's own is necessary but not always sufficient to motivate a person to seek help. Additionally, there must be an expectation that a solution is possible; in short, there must be both anxiety and hope. If a person does not know that a difficulty can be resolved, she will seldom define it as a problem. Rather, it may be referred to as "just a part of aging," or "a cross to bear." Hope can come from knowledge of human services and the expectation that professionals can be of assistance.

FEAR AND OTHER BARRIERS TO ASSISTANCE

For many persons, late life is the first time they have encountered problems (other than illness) that they cannot resolve without outside assistance. If a person has been steadily employed throughout adulthood and has lived in a stable family situation, for example, she may never have had the opportunity to learn about public and private human services that assist people financially or that provide counseling. Thus, lack of knowledge of available services is often a major barrier for older persons. Research has shown that relatively few elderly persons are aware of human services developed to meet their needs and that the knowledge they do possess is very limited (Moen 1978; Snider 1980). Older persons tend to recognize only the names of programs that are well-established and national in scope (e.g., Red Cross, the United Way, etc.); the specific services provided by these groups are seldom known.

If older persons are not aware of the range of available services, they may seek assistance from whatever professional or service they do know. For example, the elderly frequently bring nonmedical problems to their physicians and nonspiritual problems to clergy. Too often, the physician or minister cannot help with the problem directly and may not be personally aware of other human services that could be of assistance. The experience of asking for and not receiving help may make the older person even more reluctant to seek help in the future. Linkage services such as information, referral, and case management have been developed to help alleviate service barriers created by lack of knowledge among both elderly and professionals. (These will be discussed later.) Such programs provide a single source of information about available programs for older persons, concerned family and friends, and other human service providers.

It has also been suggested that the elderly, even more than younger persons, feel that there is a stigma attached to receiving services. For many, "welfare" connotes an inability to make it on one's own and implies personal failure. Such attitudes among today's elderly may have been shaped, in part, by the historical periods through which they have lived (Hareven 1977). Those persons now reaching retirement age will be the last generation with personal memories of public assistance prior to the Social Security Act of 1935. Many members of this and older cohorts observed frail elderly being supported almost entirely by family, friends, and community institutions (e.g., churches) or reduced to accepting the often degrading circumstances of institutions derived from the poor house (e.g., county homes). It may be that the elderly of the future, having grown up in a period when phenomena such as self-help groups and communal living were common, will feel more comfortable seeking assistance outside the family.

It is likely, however, that the elderly will always avoid at least some human services as long as possible in an attempt to deny age-related declines and the ultimate threat of mortality. Nursing homes, especially, are so pervasively thought of as "a place to die" that the physical and mental health of many elderly persons begins to deteriorate when a decision is made to move to such an institution at a date in the near future (Tobin & Lieberman 1976). It has been repeatedly demonstrated that most older people fear dependency more than they fear death, and will deny evidence of their own aging in spite of overwhelming evidence. One study, for example, found that one-third of persons over the age of seventy defined themselves as "middle-aged" (Bultena & Powers 1978).

The desire to maintain control over one's circumstances and a sense of one's self as a competent adult is often expressed indirectly. For example, human service providers encounter elderly persons who could continue to function independently by moving to an apartment complex where group meals and housekeeping services are available. However, it is common for these elderly to resist strongly the idea of giving up the house in which they lived most of their lives as competent wage-earners, parents, and citizens. Similarly, the elderly often refuse to spend the "nest egg saved for a rainy day" even to obtain services that would allow them to remain independent.

Self-created service barriers such as these can be difficult to address because they also serve an important psychological function for the individuals involved. Research findings have suggested that older persons who continue to define themselves as competent adults may actually remain so longer than some of their peers. In a Bultena and Powers (1978) study, persons who came to define themselves as elderly or old during a ten-year period after age seventy were more likely to die during the same time period.

Finally, services are often requested for the elderly by other persons: family members, concerned friends, and the like. Requests from others are usually based on genuine concern about the older person, but do not necessarily correspond to the potential clients' view of their own situation. To complicate matters, the elderly will sometimes initially go along with the referral to avoid offending their concerned relatives or friends, and the service provider may be unaware that they do not believe professional assistance is necessary. If the client and service provider do not agree that a problem exists or on what the nature of the difficulty is, there is very little chance that their work together will have a successful outcome.

HELPING AN OLDER PERSON BECOME A CLIENT

How, then, can providers help older persons make use of human services that could alleviate their difficulties? Probably the most common barrier created by professionals is forgetting that, at the point of first contact with an agency, elderly individuals are not yet clients. Rather, they are applicants who must make a conscious decision to accept the role of client (Perlman 1968).

The process by which an applicant becomes a client has received insufficient attention by professionals. One recent model of social service identifies four separate decisions that must be made in this process (Specht 1988; Specht & Specht 1986). Before an elderly person can be considered a client of a given agency or provider there must be

1. determination of need,

2. establishment of eligibility,

3. assessment of personal resources, and

4. negotiation of a contract

At each of these decision points, several outcomes are possible. The process may be terminated due to a negative decision; the applicant may be referred to another, more appropriate provider; or a positive decision may lead either to the next decision point or to service provision. It is of utmost importance to remember that the applicant, as well as the provider, may decide against service at any point in the process. (Sufficient attention is seldom given to this issue, even in the model being described here.)

Let us return to Ms. G. and the nurse for examples of the decisions required to establish a client/provider relationship. First, the provider and the applicant must determine that the agency does provide services that can meet the applicant's need. If the clinic lacks an orthopedic specialist, it will not be able to provide treatment for arthritis. In this case, the, the nurse should provide Ms. G. with information about other clinics or providers who would be better equipped to assist her. The process may also terminate at this point if available services do not match Ms. G.'s definition of her need. Perhaps, for example, Ms. G. does not view arthritis as a "treatable" illness but, rather, as a part of aging that leads to dependence on others. In this case, the applicant may be seeking homemaker services that are not available through the clinic. If the nurse cannot provide information that changes Ms. G.'s perspective on arthritis, the applicant may choose not to pursue services that are available such as medical assessment, medications, and physical therapy. In this situation as well, the nurse should provide Ms. G. with information about agencies that do render homemaker services.

If the clinic to which Ms. G. is applying is publicly funded, it may require that users be of a certain age, fall below a particular income level, or live in a defined geographic area of the city. The nurse must determine whether Ms. G. meets these eligibility requirements before spending too much time assessing her problem and raising her hopes unrealistically. Ms. G., for her part, must decide whether she is willing to pay the "cost" of passing this first hurdle. For example, she might feel that her finances are a personal matter and that divulging the required information is a greater infringement on her privacy and pride than she is willing to tolerate.

Once need and eligibility have been established, provider and applicant must assess whether the potential client's personal resources are adequate and appropriate for accepting a client role. Funding for human services is too often insufficient to meet existing needs, and providers decide which applicants will receive scarce services. Such dilemmas are frequent in health care, especially when specialized and costly technology is involved. Let us assume that Ms. G. has applied to this particular clinic because it has a knee joint replacement program. Not only may this program limit the number of clients it can accept, but it may also impose additional requirements to assure that those accepted have a high probability of successful surgical outcome. Clients might be required to be in good health other than their arthritic difficulties, thus lessening the chances of adverse effects from surgery and anesthesia.

Ms. G. will also have to weigh the costs to her personal resources against the potential benefits to be received. The procedure may be expensive and, if it is defined as experimental, she will not be reimbursed by Medicare or other insurance policies. Information about the amount of pain she is likely to experience and the length of time required for recovery will also have to be weighed. Since only the applicant knows what she will have to forego to meet these costs (purchases, vacations, special family events), only she is in a position to determine whether the ultimate benefits of becoming a client are of sufficient value.

Finally, if the applicant and the provider have made positive decisions at all other points, a contract must be negotiated that is acceptable to both of them. Whether it is written or verbal, this contract should attempt to specify clearly what will be asked of the client and what services will be provided. It is often more difficult than it first appears to inform an applicant fully about the experience she is agreeing to undertake. Pain, for example, is as much subjective as objective; people are sometimes surprised by the intense discomfort of a medical procedure that they had been told would be "uncomfortable." If the service is of a type that has not been received in the past, the client may be ill-equipped to translate a verbal description into an anticipated experience. If Ms. G. has never before had any surgery, she may lack a frame of reference to understand statements about the degree of pain this procedure will entail or to appreciate the depth and length of the postsurgical fatigue she is told to expect.

Such communication problems are often compounded when a service can be provided in different ways. If Ms. G. is offered "counseling" to help her adjust to the realities of arthritis, she may be consenting to discuss new ways of doing things or to allow deep fears to surface and be experienced. Providers must make every effort to explain in advance what the client is likely to experience and to obtain mutual agreement to work together, not just in a general, but in a particular way. Even after the service is accepted and begun, periodic inquiries should be made about the client's experience, and allowance should be made for contract renegotiations.

Full attention to mutual agreement at all decision points is an ethical responsibility not only of human service providers but of the client as well. Client/provider agreement on the problem and its preferred solution has been shown to be vital to successful service outcome. In counseling programs, for example, up to two-thirds of applicants do not return for a second appointment (Perlman 1968). Common explanations for this phenomenon include lack of clarity in the applicant's understanding and expectations, unresponsiveness of the provider to the applicant's needs and expectations, and lack of mutual planning to meet the client's need (Mayer & Timms 1970; Shyne 1957).

There is one other provider mistake that can forestall the process of becoming a client. Many human service providers are appropriately aware that their relationship with clients is important in any healing process. However, they make the mistake of assuming that the first task with a new client is "to establish a relationship." The problems with this perspective are twofold. First, to concentrate on relationship building is to ignore the fact that the applicant must agree to take on a client role and that that decision must be based on information gathered in the first meetings. Simply put, an applicant cannot develop a relationship with a provider before deciding to become a client.

Additionally, any relationship formed before client and provider decide to work together is necessarily different from the relationship that can be formed in the process of working together on a problem. When a provider first meets an applicant, attempts are made to maintain a tone that is friendly, sympathetic, and conveys the desire to help. These elements will continue after the applicant becomes a client, but may be mixed with firmness and insistence on dealing with issues that the client would rather avoid. The initial information-gathering and decision-making process must necessarily be conducted in accordance with social norms for conduct among strangers and one might say that these exchanges entail a type of relationship.

But the relationship that assists in problem solving and healing is much deeper and more hard won. A "therapeutic relation" can only develop from the sometimes difficult and emotional process in which two people engage to resolve the problems of one of them (the client). It is based on the clients' experience of being understood, accepted, and supported when they are at their most vulnerable. Such relationships are probably present to a degree in all human services and, in some cases, are essential to providing effective assistance. But they require their own time and attention and cannot be substituted for assisting someone through the process of deciding to become a client (Perlman 1979).

TEAM APPROACHES TO GERIATRIC SERVICES

Many professions involved in services to the elderly have traditionally been organized in independent practices (e.g., physicians) or in agencies devoted to a specific human need (e.g., social workers in financial assistance programs). Such service models are increasingly considered ineffective for dealing with the multiple, interacting problems typical of elderly clients.

As people age, a variety of physical, emotional, and social factors take their toll on health, vitality, and ability to function independently. Persons aged seventy-five and over, especially, tend to have chronic, complex problems that necessitate both medical and social services (Berkman, Campion, Swagerty & Goldman 1983). Physical, emotional, and cognitive disorders can all affect functional health and the ability to follow prescriptions for self-care. Difficulties with personal care can, in turn, lead to new health problems. For example, poor ambulation can increase the risk of injuries from falls, and an inability to leave one's house can lead to depression. Both elderly patients and their family members may need emotional and/ or financial support to deal with stresses created by illness. Psychosocial aspects of illness are especially critical in geriatric services, given the chronic nature of many late-life diseases, the fixed incomes of most elderly, and the large numbers of elderly who live alone.

Even identifying the cause of an older person's difficulties can be difficult. Several studies have found that as many as 65 percent of physically ill geriatric patients also have psychiatric problems (Whanger 1980). As many as 24 percent of older patients in psychiatric settings have been found to have predominantly medical problems, while 34 percent of elderly patients in medical settings have primarily psychiatric problems (Kidd 1962).

Many factors account for the complexities of diagnoses of elderly patients. For example, physical illness may produce different symptoms in the elderly than in younger adults, including some symptoms that are usually associated with psychiatric disorders. Depression, confusion, and memory loss can be produced by such diverse physical disorders as congestive heart failure, malnutrition, anemia, infection, cardiovascular accident, pulmonary disease, head trauma, tumor, metastatic carcinoma, postoperative and post-traumatic syndrome, Parkinson's disease, metabolic imbalance, and vitamin deficiency or depletion. Both prescription and over-the-counter medications can cause problems for the elderly, among them depression, confusion, irritability, memory impairment, apathy, and sluggishness. Additionally, older persons often describe symptoms that usually indicate physical illness when the disorder is actually psychiatric. Depression, especially, is often misdiagnosed in older persons who may complain of stomach pains rather than feeling sad.

It has been argued that the multifaceted and interactive nature of physical, emotional, and social problems in the elderly demands a multidisci-plinary approach to assessment and treatment (Berkman, Campion, Swager-ty & Goldman 1983; Clarfield & Davis 1984; Gerner 1979; Hoffman 1984; Kleh, Lange, Karu & Amos 1978; Pfieffer, 1980). Human services for the elderly must include long-term monitoring of physical and mental health, activities of daily living, social functioning, and economic resources. To meet these multiple care needs, multidisciplinary teams are needed whose members include internists, psychiatrists, nurses, psychologists, social workers, and other allied-health professionals. All professionals on the team need special geriatric training.

The team approach to geriatric services is widely considered to be the preferred mode of practice (Beckhard 1972). In the ideal situation, permanent teams composed of core professionals (physicians, nurses, social workers, and sometimes others) make home visits as a routine part of assessing the elderly person's problems and needs. The same team provides services to the client, obtains the services of other professionals as necessary, and records changes in the client's status over time. Thus, not only can various services be coordinated, but the elderly person can maintain contact with familiar providers and develop trust in their opinions, thereby easing referrals to other specialists.

Given all the advantages of team practice, one might ask why it is not more common. There is much more involved in this approach to serving the elderly than simply collecting a group of providers in one place. Team practice is complex and sometimes difficult, though often well worth the effort.

Definitions of Team Practice

Attempts to define team practice often bog down in semantic debates. A variety of terms have been used to differentiate professional teams (Ducanis & Golin 1979). When a team is composed of several members of the same profession, it may be referred to as an "intraprofessional" or "intradisciplinary" team. The status and skill levels of these team members may differ. For example, mixed teams of social welfare personnel (M.S.W., B.S.W., and case aide) have been used in both the United States and the United Kingdom to provide services to the elderly (Brieland, Briggs & Leuenberger 1973; Parsloe 1981). More commonly, human service teams are composed of members from different professions. These have been described as "multidisciplinary," "transdisciplinary," "interprofessional," and "interdisciplinary."

Each of these terms is useful in specific situations. However, only two distinctions are immediately relevant to current geriatric practice. Given the multiple nature of problems facing the elderly, any agency serving that population will necessarily involve some sort of *multidisciplinary* team. That is, a variety of professions must be potentially available either as agency staff or through consultative or referral arrangements. Collecting experts in and of itself, however, is not sufficient for optimal service. Team members must develop comfortable and effective ways of working together and sharing their specific knowledge and skills. The further a multidisciplinary team has evolved as a working group, the more it can be said to engage in *interdisciplinary* practice.

How Teams Function

There are many different types of teams and each operates differently on a day-to-day basis. However, all teams have in common certain characteristics of composition and functions (Ducanis & Golin 1979).

A team consists of two or more individuals working in collaboration. Teams may be as small as a pair of providers (e.g., a nurse and a social worker) or they may be as large as the entire staff of an agency and include all professionals whose expertise may be needed by some client. Usually, at least one team member is a degreed professional; other team members may be professionals, paraprofessionals, or volunteers. A primary purpose of human service teams is to coordinate the input of these diverse experts to provide the best service possible to their elderly clients. Toward that end, the team is a "collaborative endeavor whereby the diverse skills and expertise of team members are combined to provide solutions to specific problems" (Ducanis & Golin 1979).

Teams may operate through face-to-face or non-face-to-face interactions. Many teams meet regularly as a group; however, there are teams whose members rarely or never meet face-to-face. Instead, they may communicate through written materials, telephone, or radio. The non-face-to-face team is an important variant in geriatric service, one that often requires the coordinated efforts of many small agencies with specific functions. Case management, for example, often relies primarily on such interactions to coordinate services for individual elderly clients.

Teams have policies and procedures to guide their operation. These rules can range from formal written procedural manuals to unwritten group norms. In most cases, the rules include role definitions for the members of the team. For example, it is usually clear who is responsible for patient care and who will handle administrative tasks.

Teams have one or more identifiable leaders. Some teams are "leader-centered" (Horowitz 1970): a central figure exerts control based on charisma, organizational support, or professional authority. This is a traditional pattern in health care, for example, with all other practitioners reporting to and taking directions from the physician. On the other hand, teams may be "fraternal oriented," either with consensus achieved through discussion or with leadership rotated among team members.

Since a team is a small group, even when there is a designated formal leader, most actually have multiple leaders whose relative activity and influence vary among situations. For example, the physician may be the designated formal leader who makes final decisions and reports to the hospital administrators on behalf of the team. At the same time, a physical-therapist who has developed the reputation of "peace maker" may take the lead in discussions if team members have conflicting opinions about the best way to help a particular patient. At other times, the expertise of a particular team member may place him or her in the position of leader; the social worker may need to take the lead in developing the best posthospital living arrangements.

Forms of Team Practice

A team does not operate in a vacuum. Although it can be analyzed as a separate system, the team also operates within the larger systems of its sponsoring organization and its community. A variety of organizations sponsor geriatric teams: governmental, voluntary nonprofit, proprietary (profit-making), health care, educational, and social welfare institutions. The organization not only acts as a host for the team, but also defines the team's purpose, membership, clientele, services, location, and hours of operation. Additionally, the setting determines whether and to what extent team members participate in decision making on issues that affect their practice.

Teams function both within and between organizational settings. The most common type of team functions within a parent organization that provides a support system for the team's operation. This is the usual situation, for example, in acute care hospitals, hospices, outpatient mental health clinics, and day programs. Teams may also function in the community, between organizations, with staff from a number of agencies working together on a particular problem or case. For example, a case management team for a particular client might include representatives from the local Social Security office, the community residence where the client lives, and a community mental health center, as well as the client and a family member.

Teams in Institutions

Institutions serving the elderly are often medically-oriented and require the services of a very broad array of human service providers. Nursing homes, for example, are run primarily by nurses on a daily basis, but must also have physicians and chaplains available on an on-call basis. Their staffs also include administrators, dieticians, physical therapists, recreational therapists, activity directors, and social workers. Hospitals employ all of these professionals and, in addition, occupational therapists, audiologists, speech therapists, inhalation therapists, psychologists, and various lab technicians.

Not all of these practitioners are involved in any given case, but all must be available and their services must be coordinated when they are involved. Because the needs of clients differ, the exact membership of the team often varies from case to case. However, geriatric teams increasingly try to maintain a permanent core team since most of its clients will have multiple problems requiring multiple professional services. Special problems may arise for permanent teams operating within a large organization.

On the one hand, an institutional team is created by and reports to the organization that administers the institution. As such, it must follow the rules of a bureaucratic group (Weber 1947), which requires large groups of highly specialized experts, guided by detailed divisions of labor. The motivations of bureaucratic groups are impersonal, individual, and often monetary. A group of experts collected to meet the needs of a particular patient fits these requirements well.

At the same time, a permanent team is able to operate more effectively than one with fluid membership because it is also a primary group (Cooley 1909). Primary groups (e.g., families) are quite different from bureaucratic groups. They exchange services not on the basis of economic reward, but on the basis of affection, duty, or respect and out of a sense of responsibility for the survival of the group. Toward these ends, they often operate according to internal group norms that are idiosyncratic, informal, and flexible.

If human service teams have the opportunity to develop as primary groups, they may counterbalance technology-driven institutions such as hospitals. However, members of teams would then be subject to contradictory norms and sanctions. They are valuable to the bureaucratic institution as individual specialists and will be rewarded for competence within a narrow range of formally prescribed activities. At the same time, they will also follow the unique norms of their (primary) practice group; they will be rewarded for this allegiance with affection.

It can be very difficult for professionals to work both as individuals and as team members. Yet it may be that resolving this dilemma is one of the major tasks confronting any team member. A preliminary team task may be developing awareness of these competing influences and their need for resolution. One may encounter individual team members who behave as if they were independent professionals, accountable only to the institutions and/or their professions. On the same team may be found other individuals whose behavior indicates complete loyalty to the primary team and its clients who either lack awareness of or reject institutional requirements. Either of these extremes is less effective than an interdisciplinary team approach that attempts to weigh both sets of requirements and constraints in any situation.

Resolving these difficulties is further complicated by the fact that most human service providers are segregated by profession during training rather than being taught to work collaboratively with colleagues trained in other professions. Thus, team members may enter a service setting with expectations concerning each others' roles and capabilities that are not based on experience. Traditional lines of authority in health-care settings reinforce professional loyalty at the expense of team building. While professionals may work within a multidisciplinary team to provide patient services, they often are accountable to the next highest person in the hierarchy of their specialty (e.g., nurses report to the Director of Nursing) rather than to the team.

Despite the difficulties, team practice in institutions can be a rich experience in which each practitioner is constantly exposed to the unique expertise of colleagues. Even in situations where team membership is fluid, each human service practitioner has opportunities to learn from many others, thereby enriching personal knowledge of the problems of elderly clients.

Teams in the Community

Most community-based services for the elderly are delivered by small agencies with restricted responsibilities. For example, a home-bound older person may receive home health care from the local Visiting Nurses Association, home-delivered meals from a consortium of churches, and be counseled by a social worker from Catholic Charities. It is not uncommon for these three providers to find themselves working at cross purposes. The visiting nurse may be encouraging the elderly client to get more rest, while the social worker tries to convince the person to attend a local senior center, and the volunteer who delivers meals tries to help by engaging the client in lengthy conversations.

To prevent such situations, many communities develop some forum in which providers from various agencies can discuss their common cases. The primary goal of these arrangements is to create opportunities for team practice. In their most formal manifestation, representatives of each local agency meet regularly (usually weekly) to compare caseloads and coordinate service plans. Even when formal case conferences have not been developed, most human service providers maintain personal contacts with colleagues in other key agencies. Informal coordination tends to be haphazard, however. Lacking a scheduled meeting, providers are often too busy to contact other agencies unless they are having difficulty with a case. Additionally, informal discussion of cases is of questionable legality. The Federal Privacy Act of 1974 (Public Law 93-579) requires client permission before information is shared among providers. Formal coordinating systems can more easily handle this legal and ethical responsibility by informing new clients of weekly interagency discussions and requesting permission to include their case in this process.

A few community agencies have been able to develop team practice approaches that are even more sophisticated than those possible in institutions. The most notable example is On Lok Senior Health Services in San Francisco, which maintains a large permanent team within a single agency. The team is truly interdisciplinary and includes physicians, nurses and nursing assistants, health aides, a physical therapist and assistant, an occupational therapist, a dietician, social workers, activity coordinators, drivers (of the center's van), and a variety of administrators and researchers. The On Lok model is now being replicated in several other cities and may become more common in the future. However, this ideal community team practice requires that funds usually dispersed among several agencies be consolidated in one program (Arnold 1988). It would take considerable time and effort for it to become widespread since major changes would first have to occur in funding for human services, beginning with the federal government.

Communities also attempt to coordinate the activities of diverse agencies through separate programs created for this purpose. The simplest of these are Information and Referral programs (I & R), which maintain current information on available services such as their eligibility requirements and waiting lists. I & R programs, in existence for almost 100 years, were initially developed to keep track of persons who were receiving assistance from more than one agency. Since the mid-1970s, I & R services specifically for the elderly have been developed in virtually every community in the United States under a mandate from the Administration on Aging. Lacking any other information, it is usually possible to begin finding out what services are available for elderly in a particular community by contacting the local

Area Agency on Aging, which is responsible for the creation and maintenance of an I & R program.

In 1978, the Federal Council on Aging issued a report that called for a central service for frail elderly, one that could monitor changes in need over time and assure that services were provided (Federal Council on Aging 1978). Such services, known as case management, have begun to appear in some communities. These programs go beyond merely providing information; they can arrange for services from local agencies to meet the needs of an elderly person. In some cases, they are able to provide services directly when what is needed is not available elsewhere. They maintain regular contact with their elderly clients (usually every 3 to 6 months) to determine whether the individual's situation has changed in the event that different supports are required.

Case management agencies are usually publicly funded, often at the state level. However, case management also has begun to develop as a form of private practice since about 1980. Most of these services are operated by a single provider (most often a social worker) or by a small group of providers. A quarter to a third have formal arrangements with other professionals to provide consultation when needed or to accept referrals for service. (Such arrangements are most commonly made with physicians, psychiatrists, psychologists, nurses, and occupational or physical therapists.) The majority charge fees-for-service directly to the client, which may be an elderly person or a family member (Interstudy 1987; McCaslin & Webber 1988).

In part, private case management seems to be a response to the concerns of adult children living in a different location from their elderly parents. Private managers often are retained as a representative of the family to monitor the elder member's situation and insure that needed supports are provided. Some of these providers are beginning to create networks among themselves to facilitate linkage among different cities and states. A family member could then call a local case manager and be connected with their counterpart in the elderly relative's community. While there is much to recommend such a system, concerns have been raised about its development in the private market, unconnected to public and charitable agencies. The fees of most private managers are sufficiently high (averaging $55 per hour [McCaslin & Webber 1988]) that they are not accessible to persons of limited financial means. Some gerontologists fear that these and other recent developments may create a two-tiered system with separate services for the rich and the poor. A few efforts are now being initiated to coordinate private and public community service networks serving the elderly.

Pros and Cons of Team Practice

Whatever its form or location, there are clear benefits to team practice in services to the elderly. The ability to coordinate the expertise of a wide range of professionals is ideally suited to meeting the needs of older persons who tend to have multiple, interacting problems. The team is better able than a single provider to understand and address the entire situation confronting an elderly individual and the family. When the services of several providers are required by an individual, communication among them is assured and each will more quickly become aware of changes in the client's status that may call for changes in the services being provided.

Additionally, the availability of diverse providers increases the team's ability to take clients' preferences into account when providing service. For example, nurses, social workers, and clergy often have similar training and abilities to counsel elderly persons about their personal reactions to health problems. The elderly to whom religion is important may be more comfortable talking to a minister, while those who trust medical personnel may prefer a nurse. If the health problem involves functions that the individual considers to be private (e.g., sexuality), a nurse is often viewed as the only one of the three providers with whom the subject can be raised. If health problems have created major financial difficulties, an elderly person may only think to mention this to the social worker.

On the other hand, an effective working team requires that considerable time and energy be diverted from patient care to the process of team building. In medical settings, where the expertise of specialists who are not part of the core team is frequently needed, constant attention may be required to keep the team functioning freely as members come and go. Since most providers are not trained to operate in teams, each new team member may have to be introduced to the idea and taught to function in a new way. Additionally, teams can only provide those services that do exist; their effectiveness will be limited by the resources a community chooses to devote to services for the elderly.

Given these constraints, it is not yet clear that team practice actually costs less than traditional practice. In a time when the population is aging, concern about costs of care for the elderly may limit the development of team practice.

Health-care facilities are one obvious setting in which to develop teams since a wide variety of specialized providers are already present and involved with the same elderly patients. Yet these organizations present especially strong obstacles to team practice. They are usually run by a hierarchical administration that expects providers to report to superiors from their own profession. More specifically, the tradition of physician as team leader is entrenched in most health-care settings. While physicians may be good team leaders, they are seldom trained to work collaboratively. Rather, medical students are typically reminded throughout training that they alone are responsible for the actions of all professionals involved in a given case. This attitude, reinforced by the reality of malpractice suits, can make it very difficult for a physician to learn to value the expertise of colleagues from other disciplines.

Team practice is probably the most effective way to meet the needs of the elderly. It is not, however, always the easiest form of practice for human service providers. Team practice requires time, energy, and work that is in addition to one's responsibility to provide services to elderly clients. But as more human service professionals have the opportunity to experience what a team can accomplish on behalf of its elderly clients, the effort required may diminish and the interdisciplinary team practice may become the norm rather than the exception.

THE EVOLUTION OF PROFESSIONS SERVING THE ELDERLY

Today, the ideal geriatric service team contains a large number of diverse professionals, many of whom have had special training in working with the elderly. Such subspecialization was not always the case, however; professions and services have evolved slowly over the course of the last century, with several periods of rapid growth. A full account of the course of geriatric professional evolution is beyond the scope of this chapter. However, several periods in recent history must be noted if the current situation is to be understood.

THE TURN OF THE CENTURY: PROFESSIONAL WOMEN

In the late 1800s and early 1900s, several new "women's" professions emerged, most notably social work, home economics, and modern nursing. During this period, the first group of women allowed to receive a college education began to launch their careers. Many felt a pressing responsibility to demonstrate the wisdom of higher education for women by making visible contributions to their communities. To a large extent, however, they found themselves barred from established professions such as medicine and the law. At the same time, the influence of the first wave of feminism led them to search for female approaches to society's problems.

Two general themes of the era also influenced the choices made by these women. First, industrialization had replaced agriculture-based society and the new social problems inherent in this stage of economic development were apparent. There was widespread concern about urban poverty, which was being exacerbated by several large waves of European immigration. Many groups of rural people sought better economic conditions through the new industries. Specific problems accompanying poverty were also seen as needing attention: alcoholism, delinquency, maternal and infant mortality, and communicable diseases such as tuberculosis. In response, new professions and human services received charitable support to mitigate the human toll of industrial progress.

A second influence came from the rise of "scientism," the belief that emerging scientific methods could be used to generate new solutions to social problems. As college-educated women attempted to create new professional approaches, their efforts often centered on bringing the benefits of science to other women and to problems viewed as appropriate concerns of women. Thus, home economics applied scientific principles to home life just as new agricultural colleges brought the benefits of science to farming.

Two of the most prominent professions to emerge from these several trends were modern nursing and social work. Nurses working in the inner city gained firsthand information on communicable diseases and maternal and infant mortality, and the impact of these health problems on entire families. Among the most notable nurses of this period was Lillian Wald, whose early experiences assisting with home births in New York provided the motivation for her career. She strengthened visiting nursing as a formal service, established the first school nursing program, and established Henry Street Settlement as a base for preventive health efforts.

Social work emerged through two simultaneous human services, settlements and charity organization societies. Notable women such as Jane Addams led the settlement movement in which educated, affluent young people moved into urban ethnic ghettos to learn from and establish services for their poorer neighbors. Focusing on social problems that affected individuals, they developed parks, kindergartens, residences for single working women, social clubs, and museums to exhibit the old-world skills of immigrants.

At the same time, other early social workers were creating charity organization societies to organize private charitable efforts and to make more efficient use of available contributions. These charity societies later evolved into "United Way" agencies as well as private counseling services such as the Family Service Association and Catholic Charities.

THE LATE RECOGNITION OF ELDERLY AS A SPECIAL CLIENTELE

You may have noticed that the professions emerging at the turn of the century focused their attention on families with children and gave little separate attention to the elderly. In fact, the elderly were among the last to be recognized by human service providers as a special clientele who required services designed to meet their unique needs.

Early social services in the United States were designed as variants of the Elizabethan Poor Laws, which had first been codified in 1601 in England. The poor law system was locally based and administered and afforded different treatment to the "worthy" and the "unworthy" poor. From this perspective, old age alone was insufficient to render one unable to work or to provide for oneself. Frail elders without family support were, at times, assigned to the poor house along with persons unemployable for other reasons (e.g., the mentally ill).

Beginning in the mid-1800s, institutions for populations with particular problems began to appear: state homes for the blind, the deaf, and the mentally ill were most common. Again, the elderly could be included in one of these groups but were seldom singled out due to age-related frailty. Mental hospitals, especially, came to house large numbers of older persons who suffered from senile dementias. At a later point in time, funds became available at the county level for support of elderly persons without families and older populations were quickly shifted to county homes (a precursor of nursing homes) (Grob 1986).

Dissatisfaction with the situation of the elderly was expressed sporadically throughout the early 1900s (Leiby 1978). The Townsend Movement, especially, had a large influence on subsequent policy developments. This plan called on the government to stimulate the economy by granting $200 a month to all persons over the age of sixty on the condition that the pension be spent during the month. It was not until the Social Security Act of 1935, however, that the elderly were universally defined as a special population who required differential treatment in many human services.

THE WAR ON POVERTY: THE RISE OF PARAPROFESSIONALS

By the 1960s, new professions such as social work and modern nursing were well established with their own graduate programs for specialized training. Medicine had also undergone a reorganization during the early part of the century, moving away from its traditional apprenticeship system and developing the science-based, medical schools and residencies that exist today. Most of the prominent human service professions were becoming internally specialized; physicians, for example, spent more years in training to become surgeons focusing on a particular part of the body than they had spent earning the basic M.D. degree.

The War on Poverty era brought large infusions of public monies into human service programs in an attempt to solve a new wave of pressing urban problems based in poverty and racism. Specialized, demonstration projects proliferated, requiring additional personnel. At the same time, considerable attention was given to creating new career lines that could lift less-educated citizens out of chronic unemployment.

One outgrowth of these concerns was the development of "parapro-fessions." The personal background and experience of individuals were combined with relatively short periods of training to create new human service providers. The hope was that these paraprofessionals could not only be trained more economically than traditional professionals, but also that they would be better able to understand and communicate with clients with whom they shared similar backgrounds and problems.

Among these paraprofessionals were physician assistants, trained to extend medical services to underserved populations where physicians were in short supply. At the graduate-degree level, nurse practitioners evolved for similar reasons. In community social services, the emphasis was often on "indigenous" paraprofessionals: workers selected to match their clients in cultural characteristics (ethnicity, poverty status, neighborhood of resi-dence) so as to take advantage of the provider's experiential understanding of clients' difficulties.

Early paraprofessional developments were closely evaluated and studied to clarify appropriate roles among diverse providers (Barker & Briggs 1968; Epstein 1962; Heyman 1961; Richan 1961; Weed & Denham 1961). It was widely recognized that indigenous providers possess attributes and skills that are of value to the human services, that paraprofessionals can be trained to provide needed services, and that the use of paraprofessionals can facilitate greater efficiency in the use of more expensive professional services.

By the early 1970s, the general thrust of War on Poverty concerns began to focus specifically on programs for the elderly. During this period, a wide range of publicly-funded, community-based services were developed, evaluated, and institutionalized: information and referral, congregate meals, home-delivered meals, senior centers, homemakers, home health aides, and chore services.

Paraprofessions were also created for many of these geriatric programs, including the use of elderly persons themselves to extend services and increase professional sensitivity to the concerns of older clients. Volunteers of all ages also became important in many programs for the elderly (McCaslin 1983).

As services for the elderly increased, so did efforts within existing professions to provide specialized gerontological training. The lack of a geriatric medical specialty was especially bemoaned (Butler 1975). Even so, the first departments of geriatric medicine are only now beginning to appear. Other professions were somewhat more successful. In 1979, for example, there were two specialized aging programs in existence among graduate programs in social work; by 1983, there were twenty-one (McCaslin 1987).

The increase in human services for the elderly also led to the development of gerontology education as a free-standing specialization. By the mid-1980s, the Association for Gerontology in Higher Education was able to verify that 1,155 colleges and universities offer instruction in aging (Peterson 1987).

THE FUTURE OF PROFESSIONAL GERONTOLOGY

In the 1980s, economic concerns have led to a reduction of all human services, including those for the elderly. The public has become aware of the rapid aging of our popuation and has become concerned about the potential costs of providing care for their oldest members. At the worst, groups such as Americans for Generational Equity have argued that the overwhelming needs of a growing elderly population will take resources away from other needy groups, such as children, who have a greater potential to return society's investment in them (Kingson, Hirshorn & Cornman 1986).

On the other hand, awareness of the growing elderly population has led to recognition that more human service providers must be trained in gerontology to meet future needs. A widely disseminated Bureau of Labor Statistics report estimated that there will be 700,000 new jobs to be filled in services to the aged by the year 2000 (*Newsweek* 1982). As late as 1985, the state of California funded a special program to train geriatric health-care providers.

The relative influence of these arguments for and against increased training of geriatric providers is not yet clear but attempts to assure continued development are underway. The Gerontological Society of America published a response to Americans for Generational Equity that was sent to all public officials at the federal and state level (Kingson, Hirshorn & Cornman 1986). Gerontologists have begun to argue that the price of our past success in developing geriatric services has been an exacerbation of the stereotype that the elderly are sick, weak, and incompetent and there is a growing resentment of their public support. To reverse this trend, it is argued, services needed by the elderly must be defined in relation to specific needs rather than being tied to age, per se (Neugarten 1982).

Whatever the shape and funding of human services in the future, services for the elderly will be required along with a variety of providers trained to meet the special needs of elderly persons. As the population continues to age, professionals will also be needed who can create new, more efficient services to maximize the functioning and maintain the dignity of our elders. The field of human services for the elderly is still in its infancy and awaiting further development by new generations of providers.

FOR DISCUSSION

1. What human services can you think of that do not exist, as far as you are aware, but that might be helpful to the elderly?
2. When elderly persons are reluctant to use a service that is unfamiliar to them, what may they fear? What might they imagine will happen to them if they use the service?
3. In your own experience, what kinds of problems can arise when people who have different points of view try to work together? What approaches are helpful in working through these differences?
4. How might services for the elderly differ if they are provided by professionals who do or do not have special training in working with the aged?

REFERENCES

Arnold, M. Diane. "Covering the Uncovered: Issues and Challenges in Financing and Organizing Long-Term Care for the Elderly in the United States." Unpublished doctoral dissertation, The University of California at Berkeley, The School of Social Welfare, 1988.

Barker, Robert L., and Briggs, T. L. *Differential Use of Social Work Manpower.* New York: National Association of Social Workers, 1968.

Beckhard, R. "Organizational Issues in Team Delivery of Comprehensive Health Care." *Milbank Memorial Quarterly* 1972 (July 1): 287-316.

Berkman, Barbara, Campion, E. W., Swagerty, E., and Goldman, M. "Geriatric Consultation Team: Alternate Approach to Social Work Discharge Planning." *Journal of Gerontological Social Work* 5, no. 3, (1983): 77-88.

Brieland, Donald, Briggs, T., and Leuenberger, P. *Team Model of Social Work Practice.* Syracuse University: Manpower monograph, Number 5, 1973.

Bultena, G. L. and Powers, E. A. "Denial of Aging: Age Identification and Reference Group Orientations." *Journal of Gerontology* 33, no. 5 (1978): 748-754.

Busse, Ewald W. "Old age." In S. I. Greenspan and G. H. Pollock (eds.), *The Course of Life: Psychoanalytic Contributions toward Understanding Personality Development.* (Vol. III: Adulthood and the Aging Processes.) Bethesda, Md.: National Institute of Mental Health, 1980.

Butler, Robert N. *Why Survive? Being Old in America.* New York: Harper and Row, 1975.

Clarfield, A. M., and Davis, Sir Mortimer B. "Multidisciplinary Teams: Common Goals and Communications." *Clinical Gerontologist* 2, no. 2 (1984): 38-40.

Cooley, C. H. *Social Organization.* New York: Scribner's, 1909.

Epstein, Laura. "Differential Use of Staff: A Method to Expand Social Services." *Social Work* 7 (1962): 66-72.

Federal Council on Aging. *Public Policy and the Frail Elderly.* Washington, D.C.: U.S. Department of Health, Education, and Welfare, Office of Human Development, 1978.

Finkel, S., et al. *The 1981 White House Conference on Aging: Task Force Report of the American Psychiatric Association.* Washington, D.C.: American Psychiatric Association, 1981.

Germain, Carole, and Gitterman, Alex. *The Life Model of Social Work Practice.* New York: Columbia University Press, 1980.

Gerner, R. H. "Depression in the Elderly." In O. J. Kaplan (ed.), *Psychopathology of Aging.* New York: Academic Press, 1979.

Golant, Stephen M., and McCaslin, Rosemary. "A Functional Classification of Services for Older People. *Journal of Gerontological Social Work* 1, no. 3 (1979): 187-210.

Grob, Gerald N. "Explaining Old Age History." In D. Van Tassel and P. N. Stearns (eds.), *Old Age in a Bureaucratic Society.* New York: Greenwood, 1986.

Hareven, Tamara K. "Family Time and Historical Time." *Daedalus* 106 (1977): 57-70.

Heyman, M. M. "Criteria for the Allocation of Cases According to Levels of Staff Skill." *Social Casework* 42, no. 7 (1961): 325-331.

Hoffman, R. S. "Operation of a Medical-Psychiatric Unit in a General Hospital Setting." *General Hospital Psychiatry* 6 (1984): 93-99.

Horowitz, J. *Team Practice and the Specialist: An Introduction to Interdisciplinary Teamwork.* Springfield, Ill.: Charles Thomas, 1970.

Interstudy, Center for Aging and Long Term Care. *Private Case Management for Older Persons and Their Families.* Excelsior, Minn.: Interstudy (July 1987).

Kaplan, Oscar J. "Introduction." In O. J. Kaplan (ed.), *Psychopathology of Aging.* New York: Academic Press, 1979.

Kidd, C. B. "Misplacement of the Elderly in Hospital." *British Medical Journal* 2 (1962): 1491-1495.

Kingson, Eric R., Hirshorn, Barbara A., and Cornman, John M. *Ties that Bind: The Interdependence of Generations.* Washington, D.C.: Seven Locks Press, 1986.

Kleh, J., Lange, P., Karu, E., and Amos, C. "Differential Diagnosis of the Disturbed Elderly Patient. *Hospital and Community Psychiatry* 29, no. 11 (1978): 735-738.

Kramer, M., Taube, C. A., and Redick, R. W. "Patterns of Use of Psychiatric Facilities by the Aged: Past, Present, and Future." In C. Eisdorfer and M. P. Lawton (eds.), *Psychology of Adult Development and Aging.* Washington, D.C.: American Psychological Association, 1973.

Krout, John A. "Knowledge and Use of Service by the Elderly: A Critical Review of the Literature." *International Journal of Aging and Human Development* 17 (1983): 153-167.

Leiby, James. *A History of Social Welfare and Social Work in the United States.* New York: Columbia University Press, 1978.

Mayer, John E., and Timms, Noel. *The Client Speaks.* New York: Atherton Press, 1970.

McCaslin, Rosemary. "Service Utilization by the Elderly: The Importance of Orientation to Formal System." *Journal of Gerontological Social Work,* 11, no. 1 (1989).

———. *The Older Person as a Mental Health Worker.* New York: Springer, 1983.

———. "Reframing Research on Service Use among the Elderly: An Analysis of Recent Findings." *The Gerontologist* 30, no. 1 (1975).

———. "Substantive Specialization in Master's Level Social Work Curricula." *Journal of Social Work Education* 23, no. 2 (1987): 8-18.

McCaslin, Rosemary, and Calvert, Welton R. "Social Indicators in Black and White: Some Ethnic Considerations in Delivery of Service to the Elderly." *Journal of Gerontology* 30, no. 1 (1975): 60-66.

McCaslin, Rosemary, and Webber, Pamela A. "Social Workers in Private Geriatric Case Management Agencies: A Challenge to Social Work Education." Paper presented at the Annual Program Meeting of the Council on Social Work Education, Chicago, Ill., March, 1989.

Moen, Elizabeth. "The Reluctance of the Elderly to Accept Help." *Social Problems* 25 (1978): 293-303.

Neugarten, Bernice L. (ed.) *Age or Need? Public Policies for Older People.* Beverly Hills: Sage, 1982.

Newsweek staff. "Growth of Industries of the Future." *Newsweek* (October 18, 1982-83).

Parsloe, P. *Social Service Area Teams.* London: George Allen and Unwin, 1981.

Perlman, Helen H. *Persona: Social Role and Personality.* Chicago: University of Chicago Press, 1968.

———. *Relationship: The Heart of Helping People.* Chicago: The University of Chicago Press, 1979.

Peterson, David A. "Gerontology Courses." *AGHE/USC National Survey of Gerontology Instruction.* Report No. 4, Spring, 1987.

Pfeiffer, Eric. "Psychopathology and Social Pathology." In J. E. Birren and K. W. Schaie (eds.), *Handbook of the Psychology of Aging.* New York: Van Nostrand Reinhold, 1977.

———. "The Psychosocial Evaluation of the Elderly Patient." In E. W. Busse and D. G. Blazer (eds.), *Handbook of Geriatric Psychiatry.* New York: Van Nostrand Reinhold, 1980.

Richan, W. C. "A Theoretical Scheme for Determining Roles of Professional and Nonprofessional Personnel." *Social Work* 6, no. 4 (1961): 22-28.

Shanas, Ethel, and Maddox, George L. "Aging, Health, and the Organization of Health Resources." In R. H. Binstock and E. Shanas (eds.), *Handbook of Aging and the Social Sciences.* New York: Van Nostrand Reinhold, 1976.

Shyne, Ann W. "What Research Tells Us About Short-Term Cases in Family Agencies." *Social Casework* 38, no. 5 (1957): 223-231.

Snider, Earle L. "Awareness and Use of Health Services by the Elderly: A Canadian Study." *Medical Care* 18, no. 12 (1980): 1177-1182.

Specht, Harry, and Specht, Riva. "Social Work Assessment: Route to Clienthood." *Social Casework* 67, nos. 10 and 11 (1986): 525-532, 587-593.

Specht, Harry. *New Directions for Social Work Practice.* Englewood Cliffs, N.J.: Prentice Hall, 1988.

Tobin, Sheldon S., and Lieberman, Morton A. *Last Home for the Aged.* San Francisco: Jossey-Bass, 1976.

Weber, Max. *The Theory of Social Economic Organization.* (A. M. Henderson and T. Parsons, eds. and trans.) New York: Oxford, 1947.

Weed, and Denham, W. H. "Toward More Effective Use of the Nonprofessional Worker: A Recent Experiment. *Social Work,* 4, no. 6 (1961): 29-36.

Whanger, A. D. "Treatment Within the Institution." In E. W. Busse and D. G. Blazer (eds.), *Handbook of Geriatric Psychiatry.* New York: Van Nostrand Reinhold, 1980.

Zarit, Steven H. *Aging and Mental Disorders: Psychological Approaches to Assessment and Treatment.* New York: The Free Press, 1980.

7

The Purpose and Meaning of Activities

Richelle N. Cunninghis

Early workers, often only half-jokingly, referred to activity programs in their facilities as the BBC: bingo, bowling, and crafts. Most programs have come a long way since then, and the word "activity," as defined by activities personnel today, means "anything that a person does during his or her waking hours that is not treatment." With the use of this definition, the scope is broadened greatly, and it is possible to see that many things can be classified as "activity" in addition to leisure and recreational pursuits. The performance of housekeeping or activities-of-daily-living (ADL) functions, and work roles (actions that require responsibility and are task-oriented) are the two other major categories that also meet these criteria.

It is important to recognize that, as implied in our definition, "activity" is not going on only when provided or supervised by activities personnel. Too often, residents are spoken of as "not doing anything," because they do not participate in formal, organized activities. Actually, the ideal residents become independent recreators; that is, they take responsibility for the fulfillment of their own needs and interests, as most of us do. The role of the activities staff is to help identify what these needs and interests are and then to help devise ways in which residents can meet them given present surroundings.

These surroundings are also a prime concern of activities personnel. Although no facility can ever simulate a home environment, it is part of administration's responsibility to help provide as stimulating and comfortable a setting as possible within the confines of an institution. This includes

151

ease of access to such things as cards, puzzles, magazines, newspapers, etc., and reality props such as clocks, calendars, and pictures being very much in evidence. Also, chairs should be arranged in a manner conducive to socialization, not lined up against the walls, in rows, or in front of a television set that no one is watching.

"Environment" also refers to people and their attitudes toward the residents: the activity staff often makes the least demands on the residents and is thus most likely to be available to listen to personal concerns. Activities people do not have to give medications or examinations and are often aware of the residents' past needs and interests, and are best able to provide outlets for expressing them.

The purpose of "Activities Programming" has been defined as "providing exercise for an individual's physical, mental, and social abilities when the environment does not encourage that exercise naturally." It also specifies that the activities provided should be "of a creative, service, social, spiritual, intellectual, and physically competitive nature." The purpose of this program is to prevent or cope with the effects of isolation, dependency, helplessness, institutionalization, apathy, lowered sensory input, and atrophy.

Several states include in their instructions to those who survey and evaluate activities programs a suggestion that although some residents may appear not to be involved in activities, a closer look at their environment may indeed, show that activities programming touches these residents' lives. This is something the staff in the facility should also be trained to see.

The role and perception of the facility within its community is often another major concern of the activities department. Although every staff person has a responsibility to promote a positive image of the facility, this role seems to be part of the natural domain of the activities department. Perhaps this is due to the contact with volunteers, entertainers, and outside groups and the necessity to go to outside sources for supplies and donations. Therefore, activities personnel recognize that it is necessary to not only utilize the community and its resources, but also to publicize the idea that this is not the end of the line and that many of the residents are still capable of being productive and useful and want to be considered part of that larger community.

In order to accomplish all these goals, it is necessary to start with each individual and to look carefully at what the person *can* do—focus on abilities, not disabilities. Unlike the therapies whose prime concern is the treatment of affected parts, the purpose of activities programming is to help a person maximize remaining abilities and strengths. The following are some general considerations that may prove useful in this planning:

1. Although losses and changes are inevitable, they are usually gradual and sporadic, unless they are due to a catastrophic illness.

2. Older people have a capacity to cope and, consciously or unconsciously, do develop various highly individualized methods of adapting to these changes and declines.

3. Losses lead to deficits, but not necessarily to disabilities. Practical adaptations and the other senses can help compensate for some losses.

4. Multiple losses are more difficult to cope with than are single losses.

5. Not all older persons perceive their environment in a dysfunctional way or require special adaptations.

It is necessary for all staff to start by believing that although people are aging they are still continuing to grow and "become." The activities and environment that are provided should be designed to help them reach their highest potential in this growth process.

Specific job skills can usually be learned, but some of the personal characteristics must already be present for a person to be effective in working with older people in a program of this type. These include:

1. the belief in the inherent worth of all human beings;

2. the understanding and acceptance of health limitations, illness, and handicaps in others;

3. skill in working with people, including staff, residents, volunteers, families;

4. good organizational ability;

5. flexibility;

6. enthusiasm and willingness to learn new skills and concepts;

7. curiosity;

8. the ability to accept one's own limitations and to ask for help when needed;

9. a sense of humor;

10. creativity and ingenuity;

11. the capacity to accept responsibility and use it effectively;

12. the resourcefulness to work alone.

In the final analysis, it is not only necessary to have a genuine understanding of the broadest meaning of the word "activity" and a recognition of the importance of the environment in which older people live, it cannot be stated too strongly that a dedication to the principle that activities programming is based on the identified needs and interests of the residents in a facility at any given time is the prime requirement for a truly successful activities professional (Cunninghis 1986).

NEED FOR ACTIVITY AS ENHANCEMENT OF LONGEVITY: ELEMENTS OF ACTIVITY IN DEVELOPING SELF-IMAGE AND SELF-WORTH

Activity plays an important role in the lives of older people because it is commonly recognized that the processes of aging, both mental and physical, slow down significantly when people remain active and involved. All of the processes of aging are interrelated. An early article on activities pointed this out:

> When the individual does not participate in an adequate activity program, all of his body processes may slow down. He may also begin to experience improper elimination. His respiratory and circulatory systems may not function well, his muscles may atrophy, and the problems of aging may become more pronounced. More importantly, the patient will be faced with loneliness and boredom which in turn will cause him to become more dependent on the staff. (Comstock, Mayers, & Folsom 1971)

Activities programming also plays a vital role in the meeting of psychosocial needs of older people, including:

1. the need for belonging to a group and for companionship;
2. the need for self-determination and independent action;
3. the need for new experiences;
4. the need to be of service to others;
5. the need to be a part of the larger community in which one lives;
6. the need to give and to receive affection;
7. the need to be useful;
8. the need to have status or respect;
9. the need to maintain continuity of life experience.
   (Hunter 1955)

Entering long-term care facilities means giving up many things that are important to people and is often decided upon after a loss, perhaps of health or spouse, but certainly of home, independence, familiar surroundings, and lifelong roles. It is a time of less activity, fear of the unknown, fewer associations, and drastic change. The needs listed are not very different from those people have throughout their lifetime, but may be more difficult for the individual to meet independently, at least in the early days of institutionalization.

Companionship and being part of a group are among the most basic of needs. Although it would seem that a person entering a facility would instantly be exposed to opportunities to meet these needs, the opposite is quite often the case. It is difficult to make new friends and to establish intimate relationships; certainly one can never replace the friendships that have existed for much of one's life. By carefully matching people with similar interests and, perhaps, backgrounds, and by providing group experiences that foster a sense of identification, activity personnel can help residents to meet these needs.

Independence is a very difficult need to meet in nay kind of institutional setting. Times for meals, rising, retiring, bathing, etc., are usually set and routine; residents are often dependent on others for help in accomplishing basic tasks of daily living. Activities can help by encouraging residents to personalize their own rooms, allowing them to make as many choices as possible, while not providing more help than is needed.

The routine of nursing home life can also lead to boredom and monotony. For those who have very little to look forward to, it is very difficult to stay active, alert, and involved. A good activities program provides a whole range of new experiences and challenges and gives residents a reason to get up in the morning because there are things to anticipate.

Most people have a need to be needed and to feel that they are contributing. Additionally, many older people grew up with a tradition of service, and they want to continue to be useful and to help others. Many find ways to do this on their own by helping roommates and other residents, but the activities program can help by providing individual and group projects that will help to meet these needs by giving formal recognition for the services that the residents provide.

Maintaining ties with the community and helping residents to feel that they have not lost their previous affiliations are additional functions of a good activities program. These goals can be accomplished through

1. creating or stimulating newspaper publicity about an individual or event that might be of interest;

2. inviting the public to open-houses or special programs such as art shows or performances;

3. encouraging outside individuals and groups to use the facility for a meeting place, particularly for things that the residents could attend, such as clubs or senior citizens groups;

4. sponsoring and hosting occasions such as candidates' nights;

5. having residents participate and/or be represented in outside events as evidence that they are, indeed, still participating community members;

6. recruiting and utilizing volunteers.

The basic need to give and receive affection is often one of the hardest to meet in long-term care settings. Many older people are known to suffer from "skin hunger" because they are so rarely touched, except in the most perfunctory of ways. Residents can be helped to maintain contact with family and friends by being assisted with letter writing and calling and by ensuring them that they have privacy and a pleasant place to receive visitors. Activities that encourage physical contact, such as dancing or shaking hands, or those that involve children or animals can help, as can appropriate hand-holding, hugs, or reassuring pats on the shoulder (Carroll 1978).

Status and respect, in most people's eyes, are very closely tied to the roles that they had throughout their lives. Many of these are relinquished when entering a facility and, unlike most previously held roles, are not easily replaced by others. Roles, in many cases, provide social identity, self-esteem, and feelings of worth and personhood (Rosow 1976). Most roles have clearly defined expectations that accompany them, but there is no clearly defined role model for a "nursing home resident" and many are not adequately prepared for what is expected of them when they enter a facility.

However, there are many roles that do not have to be relinquished and, if anything, can be promoted with a little planning through activity programming. These include friend, parent, grandparent, citizen, consumer, and others that promote the skills residents possessed in their earlier years. The possibilities are endless: host or hostess, cook, storyteller, handyman, advice-giver, group member. But care must be taken to find out which roles are still important to the residents; then comes the task of structuring the schedule and environment to provide them. This also helps in maintaining the continuity of life experiences and in providing new challenges for people to meet.

Skills that are lost are difficult to regain. Therefore, the prime goal of activity programming is to help people use their remaining skills and abilities and to focus on the possibilities for growth and development that still exist. Many people enter long-term care facilities with losses, disabilities, and a recent history of social isolation and inactivity. Initially, they may resist efforts to involve them in activity because of the feelings that these conditions impose. However, once this initial resistance is overcome residents begin to feel better and to demonstrate, in many ways, a new outlook on life.

Overcoming this initial resistance may require great skill on the part of activity personnel. Motivating new residents to participate requires designing experiences that will provide opportunities for

1. helping others;

2. appropriate and meaningful activities;

3. approval and recognition;

4. successful experiences;

5. control and independence (including setting goals and making choices and decisions);

6. methods of dealing with stress and anxiety;

7. recognition of the need to change behavior;

8. rewards, incentives, reinforcement;

9. feedback, follow through, accountability;

10. improved self-concept and pride in appearance.

These factors relate to the previously identified psychosocial needs and demonstrate the important role they play in designing activity programs.

Increasingly, as people are living longer, the emphasis is being put on the quality of life. A catch phrase such as "add life to your years, not just years to your life" may sound trite, but this is precisely what is necessary if older people are to feel fulfilled, acquire a sense of continuing accomplishment, and come to see themselves as contributing to society once more. This, then, is the mandate for activities programming.

APPROPRIATENESS OF ACTIVITY:
TAILORING INDIVIDUAL PROGRAMS

All people are engaged in some form of "activity" all the time according to our definition of the word. But, in spite of the staff's best efforts, many long-term care residents may continue to resist efforts to engage them in formal programming. Men may be particularly difficult to involve because of their traditional orientation to leisure and the work ethic. However, it has been found by those who work with large groups of men that their major requirements of activity programming include an opportunity to share their life experiences and knowledge, a sense of their own personal worth, male identification, respect for their past accomplishments, purposeful and productive activities, and conveying the message that it is okay to play and have fun once in a while (Cunninghis 1986). This is not very different from what their female counterparts are looking for!

The implication, then, is that well-designed activities programs need to offer a wide range of possibilities. However, this does not mean that they are merely monthly calendars of events into which all residents can be inserted like pegs in a pegboard. All good activities programs start with assessment: the individual resident's needs and interests and the available resources (including the resident, his family and friends, the facility, and the community). From this information scheduled activities are designed and implemented.

One particularly important area of assessment is the individual's concept of leisure-time activities. What do "recreation" and "activity" mean to each person? What do they expect to gain from their involvement? What have they enjoyed doing in the past, and do they think it is possible to pursue these same activities successfully now? What interests them now: making, doing, collecting, learning? Do they like people, socializing, and group activities?

It is also suggested that the activities themselves be looked at and an analysis be completed for each activity to be included in the program. The prospective activities should be performed by the activity personnel or by someone else while observers analyze their specific components. This helps in deciding whether the activities are best performed by several people or by just one person; planning how best to go about teaching them is also facilitated. Although not all of the following observations must be written, they are part of the analysis process, which should be completed before presentation of an activity to residents.

Starting with a consideration of physical components, it's important to know if the activity requires

* use of one or both hands, other body parts;

* fine motor coordination;

* sitting, standing, moving around;

* bending, reaching, stretching;
* minimum or maximum levels of energy expenditure;

* good eyesight;

* ability to hear and/or speak;

* balance, coordination, flexibility, and/or strength.

Cognitive requirements are considered to determine if the client needs to focus on any of the following while performing the activity:

* increasing attention span,

* prior knowledge or training,

* mental skills (e.g., recall, conceptualization, analysis),

* time to learn or practice,

* creativity,

* orientation,

* initiative.

Social elements:

* Can the activity be done alone . . . in a small group . . . in a large group?

* Is there opportunity to work independently within a group?

* Does the activity involve conversation with others (e.g., staff or other residents)?

* Does it promote cooperation or competition?

* What level of interaction is necessary?

* Are there opportunities for leadership?

* What other group roles might be fostered?

A complete analysis must also include safety factors and precautions, applicability or usefulness, relevance to present life, and suitability for individual residents in terms of gender identification, past interests, identified needs, and the opportunities for adaptation for individual handicaps or limitations.

The guidelines for these adaptations would include

1. structuring activities so that residents can be as independent as possible;

2. providing opportunities to accomplish tasks *successfully;*

3. affording each resident the opportunity for *meaningful* social contacts.

In the process of deciding which activities are appropriate, individual goals are set for each resident as part of the person's care plan. If the goals are set by the resident and are viewed as relevant, he will be motivated to meet them. On the other hand, if staff have determined what the resident should be attempting to achieve, he may have little interest: good program building is a matter of identifying each individual's needs and wants, those things that are important to him in his day-to-day living.

If, for example, it is determined that a group experience will bring a resident closer to his goals, it is necessary to know, while conducting the group, what that particular goal is, not only for the individual in question, but for each person in the group. The individual goals for a group of ten residents attending a bingo game might include increasing such things as self-image, social interaction, awareness of the environment, communication abilities, personal grooming, appropriate responses, attention span, coordination, and so on.

When running the bingo game, it is difficult for the activities staff to ensure that all the appropriate residents are transported, seated, given cards and tokens, and at the same time see that the game proceeds without problems, that refreshments are served, prizes are awarded, and the like. Even more difficult is the necessity for the activity leader to be aware of each person's goals and/or needs and how to structure the group to help meet them. Each day activities personnel demonstrate that much can be accomplished, but work and planning are required.

First, time should be allotted before the group begins to review the individual needs and goals of each participant. A plan for where each will sit in accordance with his hearing and vision requirements and socialization needs should be determined. If appropriate, a volunteer, a staff person, or another resident may be assigned to assist him. Perhaps he may need to be brought in late or taken back early; comments may need to be made on his appearance; special reassurance or additional explanations might be required; appropriate rewards provided if he happens to win; or he may wish to be served refreshments if that is important. Each person's environment should be structured so that it can increase the likelihood that needs will be met: whether competition, socialization, attention span, or successful experience (Cunninghis 1986).

WAYS TO APPROACH AND INTERVIEW THE ELDERLY

As previously mentioned, the whole process of activities programming begins with assessment, i.e., a "history of life style." Assessment is an evaluation of the person's total situation, a collection of pertinent information that serves as a guide toward providing intervention appropriate to identified needs. In short, a method of learning enough about a person to tailor an individual care plan.

A well-developed activities assessment should look at problem areas and needs as well as strengths and personal resources. It should include the following categories:

1. **Medical Problems**—including allergies and dietary restrictions that may limit some activities, along with prognosis

2. **Physical condition**—level of functioning, range of motion, coordination, difficulties experienced

3. **Emotional and Intellectual State**—judgment, mental functioning, attention span, problem-solving abilities, mood, memory, orientation, social and interpersonal functioning

4. **Perception of Problems and Placement**—responses, coping devices, adaptations, expectations and understanding of illness, placement, condition, and future (and what these mean to him)

5. **Background**—social, cultural, employment, leisure, interests, religious, environmental

6. **Activities of Daily Living Habits and Performance**—adaptive equipment used, quality time preferences (*Activities Coordinator's Guide*, p. 13).

The resident may not always be able to supply this information, so other sources or methods may be necessary: family members, available records, personal observation, and the like. But even if the resident can't supply all the information needed, the initial interview is of utmost importance because it often sets the tone for future contacts, relationships, and levels of participation. The resident's full name should always be used, and care should be taken to pronounce it correctly; the activity person should introduce herself/himself by full name and title and give a brief explanation of the reason for the interview. Special care should be taken in these initial encounters to be aware of distance, height, the importance of touch, facial expressions, body language, tone and pitch of voice, and allowing sufficient time for answers.

A checklist is not the best tool to use in this initial interview, although such a list can be filled out after the interview is completed. Asking questions about the resident's hobbies, recreation, etc., may get little or no response. Here are some questions that may be more successful:

1. Have you lived in this area a long time? Where are you from, originally? Where have you lived most of your life? Do you speak any other languages?

2. How many children (grandchildren, great grandchildren) do you have?

3. Do they live around here? Do you get to see them often? Are there other people who will come to visit you here?

4. Do you belong to any organized religion? Are you active in your church or synagogue? What do you like to do with your friends?

5. Were you a member of any other clubs or groups? Have you ever held office? What did you like best about being a member?

6. How much schooling do you have? Did you attend college? What are your memories of school?

7. Women: Did you ever work outside of the home? What did you do? Men: What kind of work did you do?

8. How did you spend your time when you weren't working?

9. What did you enjoy doing with your family/friends? Do you still do these things? What do you enjoy best about them?

10. Do you read? What are your favorite kinds of reading materials? Do you enjoy discussing what you've read with others?

11. Do you like movies? Television? What are your favorite programs or films? Do you like to discuss what you have seen with others?

12. Do you like parties and being part of large groups of people, or do you prefer doing things by yourself?

13. Were you ever (are you now) interested in sports? If so, in which sports did (do) you participate? Do you enjoy being a spectator? What are your favorite sports/teams?

14. What kind of music do you like? Did you ever play an instrument? Do you still play? Have you ever performed publicly?

15. Are there any things that you never got around to doing that you would still like to try, or things that you used to do that you haven't tried in a while?

16. Do you have any special skills or talents that you think might be of interest to others? Maybe there are places you've been or things you've done that others might enjoy hearing about?

17. How do you feel about being here? Do you think you are going to like it? Is there anything I can help you with?

18. Are you having any particular problems? Are there things you have difficulty doing; anything that might affect your participation in activities?

19. How is your hearing? And your eyesight?

20. Can you get around the facility by yourself pretty well?

These questions provide opportunities to talk about the resident's family and feelings, as well as religious and community involvement. This interaction may also be the start of a positive relationship between the activities department and the resident. People in long-term care facilities, like people everywhere, are generally responsive to questions about themselves, their families, the things they've done, experiences they've had. It may be easier to start with a comment about some personal object on or near the resident: a piece of jewelry, an article of clothing, a book or magazine, family photographs, or the like. However, the most important part of the interview is the time spent in listening and in observing, which can also provide much vital information:

1. Does the resident seem to understand the questions? Does she respond appropriately?

2. How responsive is the resident? Do her replies seem to require a long period of time?

3. Does he know where he is? Is there apparent confusion about the reason for placement or the length of his stay?

4. Are there any identifiable communication problems?

5. Mood, memory recall, attention span, and apparent intellectual functioning can often be evaluated by the way questions are handled.

6. Does the resident seem to demonstrate a pattern of group or individual activity participation?

7. Does the resident display an interest in the activities currently available?

8. Are there any noticeable difficulties in the resident's physical functioning?

9. What, if anything, can be observed from the personal possessions that the resident has brought to the facility with him and is displaying in his room?

In evaluating the information gained, it is important to remember that recounting past skills and experiences does not necessarily mean that these are what the resident will want to continue to do. A person may have really enjoyed playing golf, but can no longer participate; but the important thing to try to discover is *why* they enjoyed playing golf: getting some exercise, enjoying the fresh air, being with friends, conducting informal business, belonging to the country club, etc. Golf may no longer be possible, but an acceptable substitute that meets the same needs might be found.

Once selections have been made with respect to the most appropriate activities for the resident(s), additional factors must be considered:

* approach: how best to present the activity to the resident;

* scheduling: frequency of the activity, when to pursue it (morning, afternoon, evening), duration of the activity;

* social component: individual participation, small group involvement, or a large group with staff;

* location: in the resident's room, at nurses' station, in the activities room;

* adaptations needed: resident (and staff) limitations to be considered;

* special needs: language, gender, props;

* guidance and supervision necessary;

* resources to be utilized;
* methods of evaluation;
* establishing priorities;
* assigning responsibility.

Also included may be such areas of need and recommendations to the staff as

* Give praise after each successful completion of task.
* Provide opportunities for the resident(s) to be useful to the staff and one another.
* Offer frequent reminders.
* Talk directly to the resident(s). If a participant cannot hear you, speak directly into his/her good ear.
* Encourage residents to walk.
* Give individual supervision at beginning of a new experience.
* Give constant reinforcement of reality information.
* Assist by filling in your own calendar.
* Invite each person individually.

Perhaps the most important, and often the most difficult, part of this total assessment process is the setting of goals for the individual resident. The activities are really a means to an end a way to help a resident achieve his potential, meet her needs, or resolve a problem situation. The activities can be aimed at improvement, maintenance, prevention, or coping. Goals are always written in specific, measurable, observable, and realistic terms and should require the resident to do more of something, or to do it better or differently.

Helping some residents to achieve their goals is more difficult than for others. Even when the whole process has been completed, and the right activity seems to have been selected for what seem to be the right goals, the resident may refuse to participate. It may then be necessary to look at his/her individual situation and determine what other motivational factors may be operating. As available information about a resident increases, the easier it should be to determine what factors may be affecting his participation in activities. It should be possible to list some of the general things that have been identified as affecting participation, and then determine if any of these are applicable to a particular resident.

Some obstacles that may prevent participation are:

> anxiety and stress
> lack of confidence/security
> fear of competition/failure
> fear of learning something new
> language barriers
> feeling childish or foolish
> unfamiliarity
> physical limitations
> distance from the bathroom
> withdrawal
> fear of missing visitors
> inappropriate activity

The following are some areas that may be considered useful for motivation and encouragement when trying to stimulate resident participation:

> increased self-image
> related to lifelong interests
> financial reward
> boredom
> status
> socialization
> feeling of usefulness
> others attending
> pleasing staff/family
> refreshments
> legitimate work
> relevancy.

Discovering the right key for each individual is often a difficult procedure, but the rewards are well worth the time and effort spent.

KINDS OF ACTIVITIES

Having gathered all the needed information, the next step is actually designing a program: determining what activities should be included, when they should be scheduled, and which residents should attend.

The interests and needs that have been identified from the resident assessments should be reviewed to provide the basis for the activities that will be developed and scheduled for the next month. Are there people who have indicated an interest in music, card-playing, crafts, religious activities? Can they be grouped together according to these identified interests or do some of them require smaller groups or more specialized attention? Are there several skill levels and/or functioning levels within those identified interest groups?

It is necessary to review the findings of the resource evaluation as well: the timing and location, available personnel, transportation (if needed), budget. Are the residents available for programming when the activity staff arrive in the morning? If not, should the first hour of the day be set aside for paperwork, preparation, or individual visits, or should the working hours of the staff be rearranged so that they are more efficient relative to the programming?

Other questions do remain: Are there many candidates for large group activities? Where should these be held, how often, and when is the best time? How long should they last, and who should be included? Do they require all available activities personnel or can other things be scheduled simultaneously? Can several small groups be meeting at the same time?

Perhaps, the best way to start is by scheduling one large activity every day at the time that seems to work best in the facility. Then small group and individual activities can be planned around it. A typical week should reflect a mix of spiritual, physical, mental, and social events. It should reflect the needs of all the residents in the facility, including the confused and disoriented and those who do not wish to participate in any group activities.

Once written and posted, the calendar should be adhered to as closely as possible. However, it should not simply be copied from month to month but altered continually, according to the changing needs of residents and the evaluation of past results.

The list of large group activities that can be included in an activities program is endless. Old standbys, such as bingo, arts and crafts, entertainments, movies, religious services, sing-a-longs, and parties have been time-tested and continue to remain popular with current residents.

Small groups, however, are the mainstay of any activity program. Residents with common interests can be brought together with opportunities provided to focus on the meeting of their individually identified needs. Small groups can include those formed for the purpose of reality training, games, discussion, crafts, storytelling, or the sharing of any mutual interest. Membership in clubs and on committees can offer many valuable benefits to the residents. In additon to the continuation of past interests and skills, they offer opportunities for

independence
purpose
sociability
decision making
friendships
learning about self/others
fun and enjoyment
increased communication skills
expressing creativity
sense of participation.

Committees are groups formed to perform a function or to establish policy, either on an ad hoc or ongoing basis. They can be established to serve specific needs of the facility such as activity selection, welcoming new residents, party planning, filling religious needs, education, "sunshine" (cheering up the sick or sad), or clean-up.

On the other hand, clubs are groups of persons who share common interests: cooking, gardening, photography, music appreciation, collecting (of any type), nature, travel, politics, or past organizational affiliations (Elks, Knights of Columbus, Freemason, etc.). However, it is not always safe to assume that a common interest will assure compatibility among group members. It is necessary to determine how each person's interest is manifested, and measure his/her current level of involvement, functioning, and socialization skills.

The last area of planning and preparation to be considered focuses on activities for the individual. Too often, those residents who are identified as not being able or willing to participate in groups are seen on an irregular basis, at best, and little thought is put into what their activity program should be.

The process for selecting individual activities should be the same as that for groups. Starting with the person's identified needs and interests, a program should be set up that will help to satisfy them. Hit-or-miss visits by activities personnel who have a few minutes is simply not enough. Goals and plans should be scheduled for staff to visit and discuss residents' concerns. Additionally, the staff should make sure that any necessary materials are provided, independent functioning is being encouraged, and that each resident is involved in "activities" in an adequate fashion.

Individual activities require a determination of what is appropriate for a given resident and the purpose of his participation. Volunteers assigned to particular persons for one-on-one visits should also be told what the goals of the visits should be and given guidance in the selection of suitable activities, props, or topics of conversation.

If appropriate, residents should be kept informed of other activities that are available, and they should be encouraged to attend when motivated to do so. However, as is often the case, the goal should not be to get each resident involved in group activities. Too often, activities personnel consider it is a personal failure if every capable person is not participating in planned and supervised activities. Or they worry about isolation and thus try to coax people out of their rooms who are content and able to meet their own needs very nicely. It is important to remember that group activities are not for everyone, even if the groups are small. Residents have many reasons for preferring solitary pursuits, and if it is determined that these are genuine, they should be respected (Cunninghis 1976).

"Activity" can encompass many different types of classifications: large groups, small groups, individuals, creative, social, spiritual, physical, intellectual, etc. Participants can experience activity in many ways:

1. *appreciation*—a spectator, collector, or student

2. *acquisition*—of skill, practice, improvement

3. *application*—expression, exercise, use of existing skills

4. *enjoyment*—fun, recreation

In summary, an effective activities program should provide opportunities for choices; service to others; independence; meaningful tasks; increased self-concept; new experiences and learning; use of past skills and present abilities; maintaining ties to family, friends, and community; improved orientation to present situation and surroundings; preservation of life roles; a reason to get up in the morning; and a method of enhancing each resident as a unique individual.

FOR DISCUSSION

1. How is the word "activity" defined? What three major classifications does this term include?
2. Assessment is considered the most important part of the activity programming process. Why?
3. What are three things you would take into consideration when planning an activity program for an older person?
4. How can activity programming help in maintaining and promoting the past roles of residents? Give two examples.

REFERENCES

Activities Coordinators Guide. Washington, D.C.: American Health Care Association.

Carroll, Kathy, et al. *Therapeutic Activities Programming with the Elderly*. Minneapolis: Ebenezer Center for Aging and Human Development, 1978.

———, ed. *Understanding Psychosocial Needs of the Elderly*. Minneapolis: Ebenezer Center for Aging and Human Development, 1978.

Comstock, Richard L., Rachel L. Mayers, & James C. Folsom. "Consultation and Implementation of Simple Activities for the Elderly in Nursing Homes," *Geriatric Digest* (1971): 20-25.

Crepeau, Elizabeth L. *Activities Programming. Serving the Elderly, The Technique, Part 5*. Durham, N.H.: New England Gerontology Center, 1980.

Cunninghis, Richelle N. *The Art of Documentation: A "How To" Manual for Activities Personnel*. Willingboro, N.J.: Geriatric Educational Consultants, 1981.

———. *The Activity Programming Handbook*. Willingboro, N.J.: Geriatric Educational Consultants, 1986.

Deichman, Elizabeth, and M. V. Kirchhofer. *Working with the Elderly: A Training Manual*. Buffalo: Potentials Development for Health and Aging Services, 1985.

Holdeman, Elizabeth. *A Guide for the Activity Coordinator in A Skilled Nursing Facility*. Sacramento: California Department of Health Services.

Hunter, Woodward W. "Activity Programming in Homes and Institutions for the Aged." *Nursing Care for the Aged*, University of Michigan School of Public Health Centennial Education Series No. 59 (1955): 43-56.

Rosow, Irving. "Status and Role Changes through the Life Span." R. H. Binstock and E. Shanas (eds.), *Handbook of Aging and the Social Sciences*. New York: Van Nostrand Reinhold Company, 1976.

Stensrud, Carol. "Helping Meet the Needs of Institutionalized Aged Persons." *Leisure Today, JOPER* (April 1977): 46-8.

8

Therapy and the
Professional Health Care Practitioner
Requirements and Responsibilities

Kent N. Tigges

The terms "therapy" and "activity" have wide and varying operational definitions, depending on who is defining them, be it the lay public, licensed health professionals, or nonlicensed professionals. Generically speaking, therapy and activity are defined as follows.

> *Therapy:* treatment, to serve, to take care of, pertaining to the healing art; concerned with remedies of disease.[1]

> *Activity:* state of action, quality of being active, physical motion, agility, natural or normal function, an active agent or force, social activities.[1]

These terms are general and carry no legal or professional status. Further, there is no professional or legal definition of therapy or activity that applies to professionals who treat patients.[2]

LICENSED HEALTH PROFESSIONALS

A licensed health professional is one who has been so designated by state law. State legislators study, debate, and vote on bills. If affirmative, the bill is sent to the governor for signing. Once signed by the governor, the bill becomes law, a statute. A statute pertaining to a health professional is known as a *Practice Act*. A statutory practice act governs education, practice, and, as such, defines individually, by profession, the implications (scope) of practice (treatment) and the acts, or activities used by the given health profession.

As provided by the U.S. Constitution, individual states are permitted to determine who they will license as health professionals, and they may vary in what they include in the general statute for a licensed health professional. The following, from the state of New York, is given as an example.

STATUTORY PROVISION

Title VIII of the Education Law
Article 130: General Provisions

Section 6500 Introduction
6501 Admission to a profession (licensing)
6502 Duration and registration of a license
6503 Practice of a profession
6504 Regulations of the profession
6505 Construction

Section 6506 Supervision by the Board of Regents
6507 Administration by the Education Department
6508 Assistance by State Board for the Professions

Section 6509 Definitions of professional misconduct
6510 Proceedings in cases of professional misconduct
6511 Penalties for professional misconduct

Section 6512 Unauthorized practice a crime
6513 Unauthorized use of a professional title a crime
6514 Criminal proceedings
6515 Restraint of unlawful acts [3]

The above pertain equally to all licensed health care practitioners in the state of New York. The following are specific to each health professional.

Article _____ Name of individual health professional
Section _____ Introduction
_____ Definition
_____ Practice and use of title
_____ State Board for (given profession)

_____ Requirements for a professional license
_____ Limited permits
_____ Exempt persons
_____ Special conditions

Rules of the Board of Regents: The University of the State of New York, the State Education Department:

Disciplinary procedures
Requirements for earned degrees
Unprofessional conduct[4] reference

The licensed health professionals in the state of New York are:

medicine
acupuncture
physical therapy
physician's assistant
specialist's assistant
chiropractic
dentistry
dental hygiene
pharmacy
podiatry

optometry
ophthalmic dispensing
psychology
social work
massage
occupational therapy
speech pathology
audiology
nursing
(registered professional nurse,
    licensed practical nurse)

The purpose of licensing health professionals is threefold:

1. a given professional group has a vital and essential service to protect the health and welfare of society (practice protected),

2. to assure the public, who may require a professional service, that the given professional has satisfactorily completed an authorized and accredited educational program of preparation and has passed state qualifying (board), certification examinations (qualified practitioners),

3. to assure the public that the licensed health professionals will carry out their duties and responsibilities in an ethical manner, and stand accountable if they do not.

PROFESSIONAL MISCONDUCT

Nonaccountability is professional misconduct. Although states may vary in how they define professional misconduct and subsequent penalties, the following (abridged) from the state of New York is offered as an example.

SUBARTICLE 3. PROFESSIONAL MISCONDUCT

6509. Definitions of professional misconduct. Each of the following is professional misconduct, and any licensee found guilty of such misconduct under the procedures prescribed in section sixty-five hundred ten shall be subject to the penalties prescribed in section sixty-five hundred eleven:

(1) Obtaining the license fraudulently.

(2) Practicing the profession fraudulently, beyond its authorized scope, with gross incompetence, with gross negligence on a particular occasion or negligence or incompetence on more than one occasion.

(3) Practicing the profession while the ability to practice is impaired by alcohol, drugs, physical disability, or mental disability.

(4) Being habitually drunk or being dependent on, or a habitual user of narcotics, barbiturates, amphetamines, hallucinogens, or other drugs having similar effects.

(5) Being convicted of committing an act constituting a crime under;
   a. New York State law or,
   b. Federal law or,
   c. The law of another jurisdiction which, if committed within this state would have constituted a crime under New York State law.

(6) Refusing to provide professional service to a person because of such person's race, creed, color, or national origin.

(7) Permitting, aiding or abetting an unlicensed person to perform activities requiring a license.

(8) Practicing the profession while the license is suspended or willfully failing to register or notify the department of any change of name or mailing address, or, if a professional service corporation, willfully failing to comply with section fifteen hundred three and fifteen hundred fourteen of the business corporation law or,

(9) Committing unprofessional conduct, as defined by the board of regents in its rules or by the commissioner in regulations approved by the board of regents.

(10) A willful violation by a licensed physician of subdivision eleven of section two hundred thirty of the public health law.

6510. Proceedings in cases of professional misconduct. In cases of professional misconduct the proceedings shall consist of (1) prehearing procedures by the education department, (2) hearing procedures by the committee on professional misconduct for the particular profession, (3) decision procedures by the board of regents, and (4) review procedures by the appellate division of the third judicial department, as follows:

6509–a. Additional definition of professional misconduct; limited application.

Notwithstanding any inconsistent provision of this article or of any other provision of law to the contrary, the license or registration of a person subject to the provisions of articles one hundred thirty-one, one hundred thirty-one-a, one hundred thirty-two, one hundred thirty-three, one hundred thirty-seven, one hundred thirty-nine, one hundred forty-one, one hundred forty-three, one hundred forty-four, one hundred fifty-six and one hundred fifty-nine of this chapter may be revoked, suspended or annulled or such person may be subject to any other penalty provided in section sixty-five hundred eleven of this article in accordance with the provisions and procedure of this article for the following:

That any person subject to the above enumerated articles, has directly or indirectly requested, received or participated in the division, transference, assignment, rebate, splitting, or refunding of a fee for, or has directly requested, received, or profited by means of a credit or other valuable consideration as a commission, discount, or gratuity in connection with the furnishing of professional care, or service, including x-ray examination and treatment, or for or in connection with the sale, rental, supplying, or furnishing of clinical laboratory services or supplies, x-ray laboratory services or supplies, inhalation therapy service or equipment, ambulance service, hospital or medical supplies, physiotherapy or other therapeutic service or equipment, artificial limbs, teeth or eyes, orthopedic or surgical appliances or supplies, optical appliances, supplies or equipment, devices for aid of hearing, drugs, medication or medical supplies or any other goods, services or supplies prescribed for medical diagnosis, care or treatment under this chapter, except payment, not to exceed thirty-three and one-third per centum of any fee received for x-ray examination, diagnosis, or treatment, to any hospital furnishing facilities for such examination, diagnosis, or treatment. Nothing contained in this section shall prohibit such persons from practicing as partners, in groups, or as a professional corporation nor from pooling fees or moneys received, either by the partnerships, professional corporations, or groups by the individual members thereof, for professional services furnished by an individual professional member, or employee of such partnership, corporation, or group, nor shall the professionals constituting the partnerships, corporations, or groups be prohibited from sharing, dividing, or apportioning the fees and moneys received by them or by the partnership, corporation, or group in accordance with a partnership or other agreement; provided that no such practice as partners, corporations, or in groups or pooling of fees or money received or shared, division or apportionment of fees shall be permitted with respect to care and treatment under the workmen's compensation law except as expressly authorized by the workmen's compensation law. Nothing contained in this chapter shall prohibit a medical or dental expense indemnity corporation pursuant to its contract with the subscriber from prorationing a medical or dental expense indemnity allowance among two or more professionals in proportion to the services rendered by each such professional at the request of the subscriber, provided that prior to payment thereof such professionals shall submit both to the medical or dental expense indemnity corporation and to the subscriber statements itemizing the services rendered by each such professional and the charges therefor.

6511. Penalties for professional misconduct. The penalties which may be imposed by the board of regents on a present or former licensee found guilty of professional misconduct (under the definitions and proceedings prescribed in sections sixty-five hundred nine, sixty-five hundred ten, and sixty-five hundred ten-a of this article) are: (1) censure and reprimand, (2) suspension of license, (a) wholly, for a fixed period of time; (b) partially, until the licensee successfully completes a course of retraining in the area to which the suspension applies; (c) wholly, until the licensee successfully completes a course of therapy or treatment prescribed by the regents; (3) revocation of license, (4) annulment of license or registration, (5) limitation on registration or issuance of any further license, and (6) a fine not to exceed five thousand dollars. The board of regents may stay such penalties and place the licensee on probation and may restore a license which has been revoked.[3,4]

The educational route to becoming a licensed or certified health professional is extremely varied: the minimum education being two years for disciplines such as the licensed practical nurse and certified occupational therapy assistant to four years for degree nurses, occupational therapists, physical therapists, and social workers. Medicine, dentistry, and psychology require extensive post-baccalaureate education.

THE NONLICENSED PROFESSIONAL

Within the health care arena there are numerous professionals who advocate a contribution to people in need of "therapy." These professional disciplines include recreational therapy, activity therapy, art therapy, sports therapy, adaptive physical education, exercise science, dance therapy, and movement therapy, to name but a few. Although these disciplines offer bachelor and/ or masters degrees, and in some instances doctoral degrees, they do not train licensed health professionals. This is not to imply that the nonlicensed professional does not have a contribution to offer, but that the contribution is not recognized within the health care community as an essential service that should, or need be regulated by state law. This statement does not intend to imply that there are no employment opportunities for nonlicensed professionals, or that their contribution is not of value. There are, however, nonlicensed professionals who are deemed essential and vital to health care. They include respiratory therapists, medical laboratory technicians, and electrocardiograph technicians. What is important to stress is that a prospective health care student would be well advised to investigate the professional (legal) status of a given health discipline before embarking upon an educational program.

Another issue of concern is the employment prospects of some nonlicensed professionals. Although there are health care facilities that do employ recreational therapists, activity therapists, adaptive physical education people, etc., they are not required to do so. A major consideration of employing health agencies is reimbursement (recognized as a billable service by health care plans and insurance carriers). Services that are not reimbursed are less likely to be hired on staff in our highly competitive, economically strapped health care community. One would be well advised, before selecting a health care career, to check the State Register of licensed health professionals.

THERAPY BY MEDICAL PRESCRIPTION
VERSUS AUTONOMY OF THE PROFESSION

The advantages/disadvantages, wisdom/lack of wisdom of medical authority (endorsement) of certain specified licensed health professional disciplines have been debated for decades. Irrespective of the fact that a given professional discipline would prefer to deliver its treatment autonomously rather than with the referral/prescription of a physician, it is in fact not a matter of individual choice, but rather a matter of law. Individual state statutes (practice acts) clearly stipulate the nature and degree to which medical authorization, or autonomy, is allowed or permitted. Under medical endorsement, there are two distinct mechanisms: prescription and referral.

Prescription

Prescribe: a rule of action, dictate, to designate or order the use of. *Prescription:* a written direction for a preparation and use of a medicine, procedure, or medical/health service.[1] A prescription is a specific order, written by a licensed physician, that is to be filled or carried out without alteration or substitution, unless otherwise specified by the physician.[1]

Referral

Referral: to send for, to request services or attention. A physician's referral is similar to a prescription in that it is an official request or authorization for services or intervention. A referral differs from a prescription in that it is general rather than specific. A referral may simply state, "evaluate and treat as is deemed appropriate." Whether a given health professional practices via prescription or referral, the specific document must be in hand before proceeding with the given therapy or service. Specific requirements vary from state to state, therefore, it is advised that individual health professionals become familiar with their state statute and regulations.

Reciprocity

Reciprocity is the state of being reciprocal, mutual dependence, cooperation.[1] Licensing regulations vary from state to state. Just because a professional holds a license to practice in one state does not automatically assure that a license to practice in another state will be issued. In all cases, the individual must contact the state in which he wishes to obtain a license, fill out an application, meet certain academic requirements, and/or take and pass that state's examination and pay an initial licensing fee. Once a license to practice has been issued, there is an annual, bi-, or tri-annual registration fee to be paid.

DOCUMENTATION AND RECORD KEEPING

An essential part of caring for the sick and/or disabled is documentation and record keeping. Every licensed health care agency is required by either state and/or federal requirements to keep accurate information about each and every patient's medical condition, status, intervention, and progress. Documentation includes

1. establishing the patient's diagnosis and proper coding of the diagnosis;

2. the ordering of tests and the results of tests;

3. the ordering of medications, medical procedures, and the results of medications and procedures;

4. the ordering of therapies, assessments, evaluations, interventions, and progress of the therapeutic interventions;

5. transfer procedures; and

6. discharge procedures.

Although painstaking and time consuming, documentation is essential for two reasons: (1) to assure that accurate monitoring of the patient's care and progress is appropriate and progressing toward an appropriate end. In this regard there are three check and balance mechanisms: (a) quality assurance, (b) utilization review, and (c) state surveys. The final and ultimate decision of checks and balances in regard to adequate and appropriate care rests with the state. The state agency that is responsible for monitoring health care providers surveys each health provider on a regular and ongoing basis. Failure to document accurately, inconsistencies, or discrepancies could lead the health provider to be cited for deficiencies. Should the deficiencies not be corrected in a specified time, the provider could be put on probation or even have his/her license suspended or revoked.

(2) The second reason for documentation and record keeping pertains to payment for services rendered. The majority of Americans carry health insurance, whether through a private or corporate company, medicare, or medicaid. Health insurers have specific rules, regulations, and guidelines as to what diagnostic conditions (medical problems) will be paid for and the extent of payment, depending upon whether the patient is treated in a doctor's office or on an out- or inpatient basis. Another factor that has significantly affected documentation, record keeping, and payment for services is the federal government's Prospective Payment System, which reimburses hospitals for inpatient services on a lump-sum basis. This system was developed to control hospital costs. The Prospective Payment System is more commonly known as Diagnostic Related Groups (DRGs). Based on the principal diagnosis, each patient is placed in one of twenty-three Major Diagnostic Categories (MDCs). The MDCs are broad categories that focus on the body system affected, the etiology of the disease process, the site of the disease, and any signs or symptoms. From here the patient is assigned one of the 468 DRGs based on such factors as age, sex, primary diagnosis, secondary diagnosis, and intervention procedure.[5] This complex system requires significant attention to detail in documentation and record

keeping. Should documentation be inaccurate or inconclusive, the health provider will not be reimbursed for the services rendered; the cost would then have to be assumed by the provider or passed on to the patient.

THE THERAPIST'S RESPONSIBILITIES TO PATIENTS/CONSUMERS/CLIENTS

Over the past ten years, certain allied health professionals became concerned about the manner in which some diagnostic groups were treated. It was then felt that the term "patient" conveyed an unrealistic message, that health professionals who used this term had a less than optimal expectation of the mentally ill, and the mentally retarded (developmentally disabled), and that these groups of patients, therefore, had a less than optimal expectation of themselves because they were "patients." Being a "patient" implied being sick and, therefore, supposedly reinforced their behavior to be "sick," and thus less than capable of becoming more normal in their behavior.

In the attempt to reverse this image of unwellness, two terms came into use: *consumer* and *client.* Interestingly enough there has been no evidence, to date, to demonstrate that the use of either "consumer" or "client" has, in any way, altered the manner in which professionals perceive the capabilities of those under their care, or the way that patients perceive their capabilities.

Definitions: Patient, Consumer, Client, Clientele

Patient: a person under the care of a physician, a person in need of medical care, be it physical, emotional, or social; a person receiving medical attention, as in therapy.[1]

Consumer: a person who uses services to satisfy his needs.[1]

Client: a person or company in its relationship to a lawyer, accountant, etc., engaged to act on its behalf.[1]

Clientele: the collective clients of a lawyer, accountant, etc., or habitual customers of a store, hotel, amusement place, etc.[1]

It is clear, from reviewing these definitions that there is a distinct difference between these terms. A patient is clearly a person under medical attention or care. A customer or client is a person who purchases goods or services in the commercial market place.

Health professionals have two levels of responsibilities to the public. In an increasingly health conscious public, there is a growing awareness regarding prevention. Since older adults are particularly prone and/or susceptible to medical problems as well as social and/or environmental hazards, health professionals and community action groups have taken up an advocacy position for older persons. Advocate groups range widely in their services to the elderly. Health professionals provide a wide range of information and services to the aged on how to stay as well as possible, reduce the potential effects of injury, and maintain their highest level of independence. In this regard it is appropriate to refer to clients.

In addition to providing preventive care, health professionals, by the very nature of their commitment to serve people whose health is at risk, are dedicated to reducing pathology or the residual implications of pathology, i.e., the patient in need of care/treatment. Licensed health professionals, depending on their legal scope of practice, treat people who have illness, disease, a disabling condition, or any other compromising condition that either interferes with or limits the patient's ability to function at optimal potential. Be the recipient a patient or a client, and/or attended to by a licensed professional or a nonlicensed professional, there are certain professional obligations and responsibilities to be met in working with the elderly.

There are six basic tenets for those who work or desire to work with the elderly:

1. Have regard for others.

Oftentimes older people become accustomed to sustaining old habits and ways of life and, as such, become fixed, rigid, or resistant to change. Unfortunately, older people are, all too frequently, judged by younger health professionals as inflexible and not willing to "comply" with current attitudes and values. "Older people complain a lot about their physical health, are demanding, don't listen to or follow instructions, and cause the staff to waste a lot of unnecessary time." As a result of feelings such as these, health professionals are likely to respond to, and interact with, the older person *conditionally* with such statements as

"If you get out of bed once more, I will have to restrain you, and you don't want that, do you?"

"You would be better off if you did as I say."

"If you behave and do as I say, I will let you go to the day room."

"If you would only eat better, you wouldn't be in the shape you are."

In statements such as these, there are strings attached and implications of condescendence. On one hand, some older people may fear that if they don't comply, they will not receive the care they need, be rejected, or be labeled as "difficult and/or demanding," so they submit and comply. On the other hand, there are older adults who will not submit or comply. In either instance their dignity and self-worth are jeopardized.

The flip side of the spectrum is *unconditional regard.* Unconditional regard is a genuine and sincere regard for people: for who they are as a person, *not* for what they have either done or not done in the past or the present. Unconditional regard allows professionals to care for and consider older patients under their care as unique and valuable individuals: to help them and work with them, irrespective of the elderly person's supposedly egocentric or peculiar behavior. An important part of unconditional regard is a genuine sense of respect for the dignity of people no matter what age they may be, or for the unfortunate circumstances that render them less than completely capable of meeting their independent needs. Older people are one of our greatest resources: they have made and continue to make an immense contribution to society. To ignore this is to ignore a very important facet of our own humanity.

2. *Possess a high and sustained level of energy, drive, and enthusiasm.*

3. *Acquire a high level of emotional and social tolerance for expected and unexpected situations.*

4. *Cultivate an ability to be positive and supportive.*

5. *Develop a consistent constant ability to attend to relevant and irrelevant descriptions and detail.*

6. *Possess an ease of "compliance" to patient and family lifestyles, value systems, and beliefs (ethnic, social, economic, religious.)*[6]

The second major responsibility of the health professional is to determine the patient's current level of self-esteem and to make an effort to improve it. "Self-perception" is relative to each and every person and is developed over years of personal (individual/collective) experiences and comes to be the "sense of the soul" of individuals. Self-perception is how people see, view, and value their personhood (their worth, value, abilities, capabilities). Conversely, lack of self-worth, devaluing one's self, and focusing on inabilities and incapabilities can be devastating to the patient. Self-perception is the fundamental element for self-acceptance: how a person reconciles himself, his worth and value in relation to others, and how he stands in stature to those with whom he interacts. Self-acceptance and self-esteem go hand in hand. Self-esteem is an attitude of approval or disapproval of the self. Those with high self-esteem perceive themselves as worthwhile, significant, and influential (e.g., helpful, hopeful, useful). People with low self-esteem perceive themselves as helpless, hopeless, useless.[7]

"Self-esteem is the evaluative component of self-concept, while self-concept is the cumulative phenomena of self-perception, self-acceptance, and self-esteem; it is what people come to know as 'the individual' when reflecting on another person. It can be said that self-concept and personality are one and the same."[7] When people grow older, there are continual and/or abrupt changes in their family constellations, physical environments, and/or physical conditions. It should not come as a surprise that their feelings about themselves—their self-concept—are either moderately or substantially affected. When self-concept is affected, competency and achievement toward satisfaction in life's occupational roles are jeopardized. Therefore, assessment and remediation of self-concept should be of primary importance to all health professionals. Without appropriate attention to self-concept, assessment and treatment of other problems will not be satisfactorily achieved.

Positive self-esteem hinges directly on a personal perception of quality of life. Although quality of life is relative to each and every person, there are several criteria for determining quality of life:

1. excellence of character as determined by feelings of worth and value;
2. competence and achievement as determined by feelings of accomplishment and productivity;
3. a sense of personal safety and security as determined by a substantial measure of options, choices, and control in life events;
4. acknowledgment and respect from family and significant others for past accomplishments and present/future productivity.

These criteria are essential to all people, though the qualitative measure may vary among individuals. If there is a moderate or maximum deficit in any one or more of the criteria, there is likely to be a marked impact in the person's quality of life. Subsequently, self-esteem will more than likely be compromised.

There are numerous assessment instruments available to determine patients' quality of life and self-esteem. When appropriate the health professional is encouraged to use them. An important issue to stress at this point is that all too frequently health professionals, for one reason or another, are likely to be reactive rather than proactive. In this position they use select assessments to determine symptoms. Inadvertently the problems causing the symptoms are not investigated and appropriately addressed. Therefore, treatment strategies are symptomatically treated and the vital underlying problems are overlooked. Symptoms, be they physical, emotional, or social (verbal or nonverbal), are red flags that alert the health professional to something that is wrong and that further investigation must be undertaken to determine the source or the actual problem. It is essential that symptoms, and the problems causing them, be appropriately addressed.

ASSESSMENT

Assessing self-esteem is as important in the treatment process as the assessment of physical problems. Focusing on an individual's state of mind without due attention to the physical condition results in ineffective treatment. The following protocol should be used to diagnose the presence of compromised self-esteem:

1. employ appropriate disciplinary assessments to examine the patient's symptoms (*observable behaviors*);
2. assess, examine, test *probable causes;*
3. diagnose the level of compromised self-esteem *feelings expressed.*

There are three levels of compromised self-esteem: *helpless, hopeless, useless.* These levels are hierarchal: the *first level* is helpless, the *second* is hopeless, the *third* is useless.

Helpless, observable behaviors.*

Figure 1

Observable Behaviors

1. Withdrawal from active activity due to fear of additional physical injury.
2. Excessively demanding.
3. Diminished ability to control emotions.

---

*Figures 1-9 from K. N. Tigges and W. M. Marcil, *Terminal and Life Threatening Illness: An Occupational Behavior Perspective* (Thorofare, N.J.: Slack, Inc.). Reprinted by permission.

Helpless, probable causes.

Figure 2

Probable Causes

1. Loss of physical strength and endurance.
2. Loss of independence in self care, work, leisure.
3. Bedbound/enforced dependence.
4. Dependence on medications, catheters, colostomies, nasogastral tubes.

Helpless, feelings expressed, the diagnosis of compromised self-esteem.

Figure 3

Feelings Expressed

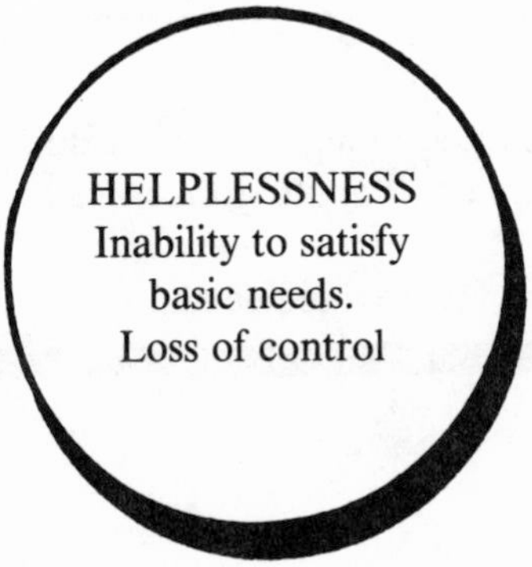

HELPLESSNESS
Inability to satisfy
basic needs.
Loss of control

Hopeless, observable behaviors.

Figure 4

Observable Behaviors

1. Anger, resentment, bitterness.
2. Inability to identify goals.
3. Strained interpersonal communications with family/ friends.
4. Increased anxiety/restlessness.
5. Excessive/psychosomatic physical/emotional symptoms.

Hopeless, probable causes.

Figure 5

Probable Causes

1. Loss of primary life roles.
2. Recognition of declining physical health.
3. Presence of nausea, vomiting, diahrrea, constipation, loss of appetite.
4. Recognition of impending death.

Hopeless, feelings expressed, the diagnosis of compromised self-esteem.

Figure 6

Feelings Expressed

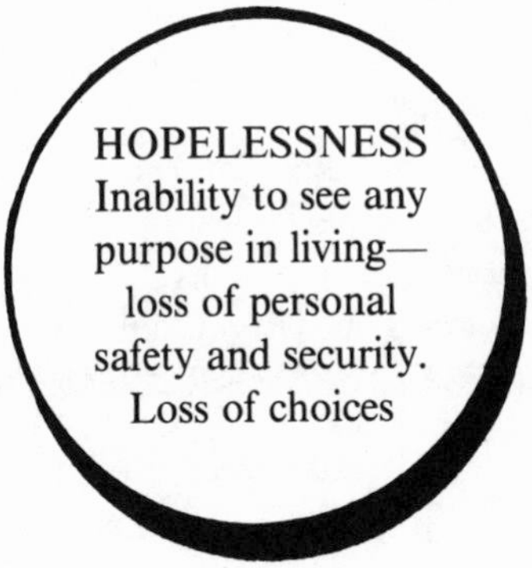

HOPELESSNESS
Inability to see any
purpose in living—
loss of personal
safety and security.
Loss of choices

Useless, observable behaviors.

Figure 7

Observable Behaviors

1. Depression and/or withdrawal.
2. Severed interpersonal communications with family/friends.
3. Imposed isolation/detachment.
4. Unresponsive/negativism.
5. Avoidance of eye contact/rejection of physical contact.

Useless, probable causes.

Figure 8

Probable Causes

1. Inability to have any direct/positive influence on immediate situation.
2. Threatened personal safety and security.
3. Loss of direction, goals.
4. Loss of purposeful productivity.
5. Feelings of being a burden on family.

Useless, feelings expressed, the diagnosis of compromised self-esteem.

Figure 9

Feelings Expressed

USELESSNESS
No perceived
personal worth
or value.
Loss of options

The assessment and diagnosis of compromised self-esteem is a key feature in determining appropriate therapeutic intervention by each and every professional. If the appropriate diagnosis is made, health professionals can put in place realistic treatment strategies to ensure appropriate options, choices, and control, which will increase the integrity of the older adult patient and her respective family members in their search for quality-of-life experiences.

The third responsibility of the health professional is bedside manner. This refers to the personal/emotional encounters that transpire between the health professional, the patient, and/or family members. When people, particularly older people, become sick, injured, and/or disabled, they are at risk. This is because they are thrown off the natural pace of their normal life routine. The chances for "recovery" and a return to their former stable and independent life routine are moderate at best. The older adult patient is not a priority in the contemporary American health care system.[8] Elderly patients are at risk because they cannot always speak clearly in their own behalf— they often do not know what their rights or privileges are—and they may not have family resources or advocates to stand in for them. When any health professional visits them at home, in the hospital, or in the nursing home, these older persons are more than likely to feel at risk. "Here are these highly trained professionals, whom I must depend on, and if I don't behave or give the right answers and agree to do what they say, I won't get the services I so desperately need."

Effective and concerned approaches to bedside manner can substantially reduce the patient's feelings of "being at risk." Guidelines for bedside manner include

1. Ability to put the patient at ease: The effective health professional is one who has the social skill to enter the patient's environment with the ease of a natural social introduction. The patient's environment, be it a hospital, nursing home, or private home, is his territory—his space— and it must be respected as such. A friendly welcoming introduction is, without question, the most effective way to defuse what might be preconceived by the patient and/or the family as a traumatic "interview" or intrusion.

2. Make casual, yet sincere comments about the patient's home/room to convey that you recognize and respect his possessions and territory.

3. Assure the patient and family members that you are not just aware of their problems but will make every effort to ease them.

4. Allow each person an appropriate amount of time to express concerns. Ill or disabled older people have much to say and to convey. Their lives—their sense of personal safety and security—are at risk; they may feel an urgency to express their multiple needs and concerns. Not always knowing what health professionals mean by "How are you feeling?" "Is there anything that I can do for you?" or "Is there anything bothering you?" the older person may "ramble on and on" about issues and concerns that may not have any direct relevance to the interest of the health

professional. The value of the time spent with a patient is a concern of all health professionals, yet economic use of one's time must be viewed, as well, in terms of short-term and long-term results. It is a known fact that if older adults are given appropriate time and attention early in their treatment, productive outcomes are more likely to be realized by the patient and the health care provider.

There is truth to the fact that older patients and their families need and request a moderate-to-high degree of physical and emotional comforting and support. There are few people who, when sick, hurt, miserable, or frightened, do not respond positively to a hug, a kiss, a gentle touch on the shoulder, or a comforting hand; these gestures are age-old, effective ways to show concern and caring. They are, however, very personal and private acts. Many people think that older people need "handling" if they are to be comforted and reassured. The notion that older people need or want to be held or touched is as unfounded as the notion that the use of first names or familiar expressions such as "Dear," "Gramps," "Honey," "Sweetie" is in any way appropriate, or that using them will facilitate a better rapport between patient and health provider. Such usage can only convey attitudes of condescension, which serves to demean the elderly.

Patient/therapist interactions must always be professional and businesslike. It is common protocol to address patients by their surnames, unless they request to be called by their given names. A name is perhaps a person's single most identifying feature and is a key component of self-concept. It is not uncommon to observe entire interactions between patients/health professionals in which the patient's name is never used. Such interactions can and do become sterile and impersonal, and patients may come to believe that the health professional is not truly interested in them or does not remember who they are or what their needs may be. Appropriate and consistent use of patients' names will convey two things:

A. that the health professional remembers the patient's name and shows regard for their individuality and personhood;

B. it will help to focus on the patient's part in the therapeutic process. Such personalization can turn the patient's attention from a position of passive reluctance to a position of positive enthusiasm.

5. Apart from body stature, eye contact can be the most powerful means of influence. It has been said that the eyes are the windows to the soul of a person. Their position—above or below those of another person—and their physiognomy can clearly convey state-

ments of superiority/dominance, concern/compassion, indifference/ superficiality. When interacting with older patients the following are suggested:

A. Following appropriate introductions, pull up a chair and place it three to five feet from the patient's face. If there is no chair, find a wheelchair or commode to sit on. If none of these items are available, ask the patient if you may sit on the side of the bed.

B. If appropriate, put the head of the bed up, prop the patient with pillows, or bring the patient to a bedside sitting position. These efforts will facilitate patient control of the situation and increase a measure of "equal" interpersonal interaction.

There are many ethical, professional and personal responsibilities that must be taken with great sincerity when engaging in practice with the sick, the ill, the injured, or the disabled. A human life is a very precious commodity, and in no way can any part of that life be taken for granted or treated lightly.

The above suggestions for bedside manner are, in the scheme of life, good and practical common sense. However, in the day-to-day care and treatment of older people, they are, unfortunately, overlooked or considered to be unimportant or irrelevant. "Who will care anyway; they are old and senile."

POSTSCRIPT

"When I grow old—I hope that I will have my health and my wits about me—because I must, at all cost—maintain my independence and dignity. After all, I have lived a long time, experienced many life events.

"I was once, in my youth and adulthood, an energetic person—who worked my best—long and hard—from morning to night. I raised a family, or two or three, if you would care to ask me about all the neighbor children, nieces, and nephews. There were good times—happy memories. Yes there were struggles, hardships, worries, and tragedies. There was grief and sorrow, yet, somehow, there was strength that came from family, friends, and even strangers. The very fabric of life, if woven well, can endure so very much.

"I am now finished with my task in life—and I sit here and wait out the time for my end to come. I am not sad or disappointed that my life will end. What does bother me, so very much, is that I have lost my health, my independence, and my wits. To me—in my mind's eye—I am just as clear, sharp, and intelligent as I ever was. Yet I can tell by the way that you talk, at me and about me, to your colleagues, that you think I am confused, odd—don't know what day it is, or if I have had visitors or not.

"During my declining days, I have had to resign myself to your care—as I can no longer care for myself. How painful it is to no longer be in the physical and emotional control of myself that I was once. I hope that you will not judge me negatively or, God forbid, as insignificant. If you could, just once or twice, think of me as a person. Ask me some questions about life and loving—and about who I am. My answers may not be clear or make sense, but the thrill it would bring to me just to be asked would mean so very much.

"Perhaps to you I am just another old person who needs to be taken care of. Please look beyond what you see and look into my eyes—please see me as the person I see in myself—and believe myself to be—please see me carefully, respectably, and comfortably to the end of my life."

—Anonymous
Buffalo, New York
1988

REFERENCES

1. *Webster's New Twentieth Century Dictionary.* William Collins, World Publishing Co., 1977.

2. Sippel, W. Executive Secretary, State Boards for Occupational Therapy, Physical Therapy, Optometry and Ophthalmic Dispensing. New York State Education Department. Albany, New York 12230. Personal conversation.

3. McKinney's Consolidated Laws of New York. Annotated, Book 16 Education Law, Sections 5501-7499. New York State Education Department, Albany, New York 12230.

4. Official Compilation of Codes, Rules and Regulations, State of New York, Title 8-Education.

5. Marcil, W. M. "Need for Alternative Model." In: Tigges, K. N., Marcil, W. M. *Terminal and Life Threatening Illness: An Occupational Behavior Perspective.* Thorofare, N.J.: Slack Inc., 1988.

6. Tigges, K. N. "Therapeutic Use of Self." In: Tigges, K. N., Marcil, W. M. *Terminal and Life Threatening Illness: An Occupational Behavior Perspective.* Thorofare, N.J.: Slack Inc., 1988.

7. Miller, J. "Enhancing Self-Esteem." In: *Coping with Chronic Illness.* Ed. J. Miller. Philadelphia: F. A. Davis Co., 1983, pp. 275-280.

8. Butler, R., Lewis, M. *Aging and Mental Health.* St. Louis: Mosby, 1973, pp. 16-18.

FOR DISCUSSION

1. Write to your state division of professional licensing and request three (3) to five (5) specific practice acts (statutes). See the list on page 173 of this chapter. Discuss the scope of practice of each discipline. How is therapy/activity defined?
2. Review and discuss the education and licensing requirements of the above practice acts. What impact might they have for those who enter the profession and for those who use their services?
3. What are the advantages and disadvantages of medical (physician) endorsement for prescription/referral versus autonomy in treatment?
4. What are the positive and negative implications of using the terms, "patient," "client," "consumer."
5. What are the implications of conditional regard and how may it adversely effect the relationship between the health professional and the patient/client?
6. Why is it essential for a health professional to have a high level of emotional-social tolerance for expected and unexpected situations?
7. In many health care centers (skilled nursing facilities, extended care facilities, nursing homes) where there is a low patient to staff ratio, how can it be justified for overworked staff to spend time engaged in bedside manner and the assessing of the patient self-esteem?

9

The Legal and Political Arenas

Connie Zuckerman

The philosophical and historical underpinnings of present American law strongly support the right of adult individuals to pursue whatever they desire, and to lead whatever type of life they find acceptable. Constrained only by the minimal restrictions provided through case law, legislation, and regulations, individuals in our society may set their life's course however they wish. Moreover, they are presumed to have the capacity to function as free and independent persons. There is a fundamental presumption built into our system of laws that all adults (defined for most purposes as those eighteen years of age or older, with the exception of the congenitally retarded) are legally "competent": that is, they are considered capable of exercising such fundamental functions of citizenship as the right to vote, to marry, to make contracts, to write a will, and, more generally, to make such basic decisions as whether and where to work, with whom to associate, where to live, and how to set the path of their lives. Society presumes that adults have the capacity to make these decisions for themselves.

This legal presumption, indeed badge, of competency does not ensure that individuals will always make responsible decisions; it does not prevent the foolish, unwise, or even irrational act from occurring. In fact, what this presumption does is to guarantee that whatever options an individual chooses will be left unscrutinized and free from government intervention, unless they encroach upon or endanger the lives of others in violation of civil or criminal laws, or unless the danger to self or others is such that it meets the criteria for civil commitment. The only valid method of challenging or rebutting the legal presumption of competency is through a formal petition in a court of law. It is only through a court order, obtained with the requisite due process of law, that an individual's badge of competency can be stripped away and with it, the attendant loss of freedoms for the individual adjudicated legally incompetent.

For the elderly, the status of this legal presumption is no different than for any other adult age group; they, too, are presumed to be competent, and are afforded all the rights and freedoms that attach to that label. While diminishment of physical abilities is a likely consequence of the process of aging, the legal presumption of mental capacity—that is, competency—remains intact unless and until a court of law declares otherwise. The elderly have the right to exercise personal choice to assume personal risk if they so desire. Yet our beneficent and, at times, paternalistic attitudes toward the elderly may belie this fact. As such, older individuals are at increased and special risk of being challenged, often through formal, coercive legal action. Despite the unquestionable right of elderly persons to make decisions for themselves (however idiosyncratic those decisions may be), it is a fact that their decisions are often questioned, if not legally invalidated, particularly regarding financial concerns and health care decisions. While it may be that elderly persons are more susceptible to cognitive impairment, that is not a necessary consequence of aging. Those who work with the elderly or provide services for them must work to prevent dangerous stereotypes from overshadowing real capabilities or trampling applicable legal rights.

Society's view of the elderly, in terms of law, public policy, and social welfare policy is nonetheless somewhat paradoxical. First, as described above, the elderly stand in the same shoes as all other adults, at least in terms of legal presumptions about their capabilities. Yet, at the same time, there is no doubt that the elderly are viewed, and often treated, differently and distinctly from other segments of society. While they may not command the respect and importance in our society that they do in other cultures (such as Asian societies), the elderly retain a unique place in our social welfare programs and in public policy planning. With age as the only criterion, and without respect to financial eligibility, our elderly are the recipients of such benefits as the Medicare insurance program, reduced tax rates, and senior citizen discounts (including reduced transit fares or lower prices on consumer items). Such programs are representative of the special, if unarticulated, obligations we as a society believe are owed to our elderly, perhaps because of their previous social contributions, perhaps for other reasons. Special government programs translate esoteric notions about the unique place of the elderly into concrete services for their benefit.

This "special" stature of the elderly does, at times, have a negative side as well. While old age commands respect and reverence from some, for others it implies the need for protective if not paternalistic behavior. Some of this bias, particularly concerns about safety, may have a factual basis. Aging is usually accompanied by increasing morbidity, often leading to greater physical frailty and incapacity. While physical impairment may mean dependence upon others for the execution of certain tasks, does it necessarily lead to mental weakness or impairment as well? Obviously not. Yet the fact of physical dependence can all too easily translate into unnecessary disempowerment: it is easy to confuse slowness in speech or movement with diminution of thought or judgment, and to dismiss the physically incapacitated elder as intellectually inferior.

To a certain extent our common law traditions encourage this easy slide into paternalism. The old English concept of *parens patriae* empowers and, indeed, obligates society to care for and protect those who cannot fend for themselves, which is usually considered to include children, incompetents, and the traditional stereotype of the feeble or infirm elderly.

This is not to say that such paternalistic actions are always wrong. Certainly they appear to be motivated by the desire to act beneficently toward the elderly. Yet such beneficence is often purchased at the cost of personal freedom to act autonomously and independently, a fundamental right of all adult citizens. Moreover, this loss of freedom often comes about without formal legal process, in which the elderly person would have the opportunity to defend herself and her rights from unfounded accusations.

Perhaps this multifaceted view of older individuals is an inevitable reflection of the truly heterogenic make-up of that group we define as "the elderly." Beyond the commonality of chronological age, what generalizations can be made about the characteristics of this group? As a whole, the elderly, particularly those eighty-five years old and above, constitute the fastest growing segment of our population. But is it accurate to label all of these individuals as independent functioning persons or, equally absurd, to compel all members of this group to a life of dependence, and often degradation, merely because of chronological age? The task confronting policy makers and those who service the elderly is to maintain and support, as best as possible, the autonomy of all those elderly who are willing and able to continue their independence while, at the same time, providing care for and preventing the abandonment of, those elderly individuals who are truly in need of assistance.

It is in the delivery of health care services, both in acute care settings as well as long term care facilities (and even in the home care setting), that this paradoxical attitude toward the elderly is most evident. There is a rich history in the law as well as in bioethical theory that elucidates and supports the rights of all capable adults, including the elderly, to either consent to or refuse proposed medical interventions, even if that refusal should lead to serious harm or to the death of the patient. The increased availability of sophisticated medical advances has forced society to consider and at times legislate whether and when the uses of such technology are appropriate, particularly with regard to our elderly population. Patients and their families have gone to court to fight for and obtain the right to decide what medical treatment is personally acceptable, given their particular circumstances. A variety of agencies, organizations, and even legislatures have promulgated "Patient's Bills of Rights," which spell out precisely what are the rights of patients, and obligations of caregivers, in the health care setting. Those pronouncements have served to heighten the awareness among those who work with the elderly regarding the moral and legal rights of patients.

Despite the availability and applicability of these rights to geriatric patients, there remains a well-documented reluctance among medical caregivers to allow elderly persons to make their own health care decisions, particularly when such choices involve risk to the patient's medical well-being. Some of this reluctance springs from a genuine concern about the patient's decision-making capacity, a much debated concept and determination that will be discussed more fully below. Some of it, as well, is the consequence of a medical school education that inculcates values of beneficence and at times paternalism into physicians in training. Whatever its origins, this ambivalence about the role of the elderly patient in our health care system continues to influence the law and public policy surrounding geriatric patient care. It is to the law, and the legal concepts and mechanisms pertinent to geriatric health care, that we shall now turn.

COMPETENCY

As stated previously, adult individuals in our society are presumed to be legally "competent." Despite the common and often casual use of the word, particularly in medical settings, the proper use of "competence" is in the legal context: it is a legal term of art. Its employment signifies a wide-ranging, global set of skills and abilities considered necessary to navigate one's course through life. Competence is also an expansive, empowering concept that grants individuals tremendous freedom, and attendant responsibilities, as citizens in our society. The legal presumption of competency may be challenged and overturned only after formal, legal proceedings. The elderly, notwithstanding any physical or cognitive impairments, are presumed legally competent to carry on their affairs. No other person, not even a next of kin, is legally empowered to act on their behalf unless a court of law, after a proper legal hearing, has declared the elderly person to be incompetent.

Given the empowerment that accompanies the presumption of competency, it is self-evident that a judicial pronouncement of incompetency can have a devastating and significant effect on an individual's freedom and autonomy. Yet it is clear that some persons, including some elderly individuals, do not possess sufficient mental capacity to carry on all of their affairs or to make all decisions for themselves. In some cases, impairment is limited to certain areas: perhaps because of short-term memory problems an individual cannot keep to a medication schedule or cannot remember to pay monthly bills. For others, the degree of incapacity is more severe, such that the assistance of a surrogate is necessary for all basic, fundamental activities and decisions.

A formal judicial hearing to determine incompetency is really most appropriate for that limited number of individuals whose cognitive impairment is significant and extensive. A legal declaration of "incompetency" transforms the status of the individual in question to that of a child in the eyes of the law. The incompetent individual may no longer be entitled to make even such basic decisions as where to live or how to spend his or her own money. Someone else is legally empowered to make these personal, fundamental choices for the person. Given the serious consequences of such a judicial determination, it is surprising and distressing to discover that in many states, the statutory definition of who is "incompetent" is vague and broadly defined. In certain states a person may be adjudicated incompetent, according to their statutes, merely if he is unable to manage himself or his affairs by reason of *age*. Unfortunately, the stereotypical picture of the elderly as feeble, infirm, or senile continues to influence the laws in many states. It is no wonder that elderly persons are at increased risk for unnecessary legal disempowerment.

The judicial process of determining incompetency requires a formal legal hearing. Such a hearing comes about through a petition to a court of appropriate jurisdiction. Any relative or friend interested in the individual's financial or personal well-being is usually permitted to petition the court. Other interested parties, including hospitals or community social service agencies, can also be petitioners. Once the court process has been invoked, notification will be sent to all interested parties, and a date will be set for the court hearing. Prior to the actual hearing, a judge may appoint a *guardian ad litem** if the alleged incompetent has no attorney to represent her and advocate on her behalf at the hearing. The *guardian ad litem* serves as an officer of the court and usually functions as an independent fact finder for the judge. Such a person would normally inform the judge

---

*A person appointed by a court to act on behalf of one who is legally incapacitated.

as to the desires of the alleged incompetent, but would not necessarily advocate that the judge respect those desires, the way a private attorney would.

During the hearing, evidence is presented to the judge and certain individuals may testify either on behalf of the petitioner or on behalf of the alleged incompetent. Very often in such hearings the testimony of psychiatrists, in addition to other caregivers, is crucial to the judge's determination. A common misconception is that a psychiatrist can declare an individual to be "incompetent." However, only judges can make that formal legal determination. What a psychiatrist can do is give an expert opinion regarding an individual's cognitive functioning, judgment skills, or affliction with a mental illness. Such a determination is often an important component of the formal legal determination of competency.

If, after a formal hearing, the judge determines that the petitioner has met his burden of proof, i.e., he has presented to the court the clear and convincing evidence legally necessary to establish incompetency, then the judge can declare the individual to be legally incompetent and can appoint a legal guardian to act on the incompetent's behalf. In certain states, the person appointed guardian is called a "committee." The judge will determine who is most appropriate to serve in this capacity and will also define the scope of the guardian's empowerment over the incompetent. Once there is a formal declaration of legal incompetency, with the attendant loss of rights and freedoms, only a court of law can reestablish the individual's legal competency.

Because of the harsh consequences of a declaration of legal incompetency, many states permit the appointment of a guardian for *limited* purposes, particularly when an individual's mental impairment is confined to certain acts or areas of decision making. For example, an individual may lose the cognitive ability to oversee her complex financial affairs or even to just attend to her monthly bill paying. Yet she may retain the cognitive capacity to undertake her daily activities and to make such choices as where and with whom to live, for whom she should vote, or to whom she should leave her assets upon her death. In such cases, courts may appoint limited guardians (often called "conservators") to oversee and manage only certain aspects of the person's life. In such cases, the individual is *not* declared legally incompetent. She continues to possess many of the fundamental rights belonging to all citizens. Rather a less restrictive legal determination is made (often the legal finding is one of "substantial impairment") by a court of law. The guardian is empowered to act only in certain discrete circumstances.

One must be cautious, however, in concluding that limited guardianships or conservatorships offer a panacea for elderly persons who have fluctuating or limited mental capacity. Despite the discrete nature of the legal empowerment and the supposed court supervision of conservatorship arrangements, the reality exists that those who control an elderly individual's purse strings often, in fact, control all other areas of the person's life. Appointment of a conservator does constitute less of an intrusion on an individual's rights and freedom than does the appointment of a committee. It stands, nonetheless, as a serious restriction of the elderly person's liberty: it is a determination made at great cost to the person adjudged to need the conservator.

The appointment of a committee or conservator for an elderly person is different and distinguishable from the process of civil commitment. Proceedings pertinent to the latter are, in general, brought about for the specific purpose of providing care and treatment for mentally ill persons living in the community. States are empowered, under their previously mentioned *parens patriae* authority, to hospitalize involuntarily or forceably those individuals whose mental illness is such that they pose an imminent and immediate risk of serious harm to themselves or others. Present-day criteria for this type of involuntary institutionalization are strictly and stringently interpreted; no one can be hospitalized under such state law provisions beyond a limited, emergency period without judicial intervention into the process. Few elderly persons are so debilitated or incapacitated that they require this type of drastic intervention in their lives.

DECISION-SPECIFIC CAPACITY
IN THE HEALTH CARE SETTING

Relatively few adults in our society, elderly and nonelderly alike, have had their competency formally contested in a court of law, or have had guardians or conservators appointed for them. The legal presumption that they are competent remains intact. Such a presumption, however, does not prevent friends, family, or caregivers from questioning, if not overriding, the choices that some elderly persons make for themselves, particularly with regard to health care decisions. The issues to be addressed in such circumstances are several: How do such questions and determinations differ from legal declarations of incompetency? How should the capacity to make decisions be determined in the health care setting? What standards should guide such determinations?

A point of clarity is necessary to begin the discussion. As already described, "competency" has a particular legal meaning representative of certain legal assumptions. Nonetheless, it is a word often casually used by nonlawyers, especially by caregivers, when describing the ability of a patient to give consent for a proposed medical intervention. Consulting psychiatrists may even declare that such patients are "not competent" or "incompetent" to give consent. These expert evaluations, however, have nothing to do with the individual's *legal* status or with any judicial determinations. More likely they refer to the given capabilities and deficits of the patient in the specific circumstances in question. What is at issue is the person's capacity to make a specific health care decision.

In the health care and bioethics literature this type of determination is more commonly and correctly referred to as "decision-specific capacity." A person may be lacking the cognitive or judgment skills necessary to decide upon a complex medical intervention yet may nonetheless remain legally "competent" to carry on all other normal activities of life without intervention or restriction.

Rarely do health care providers or hospital administrators turn to courts of law when the capacity of a patient to make a specific health care decision is in question. Court processes are often time consuming, expensive, and not necessarily able to deal in a sensitive manner with the nuanced factors that affect and influence a patient's decision-making ability. This is not to say that recourse to a court is never appropriate, particularly in emergency circumstances when controversy and conflict could lead to injurious delays. Indeed, a few commentators argue that a public court of law is an appropriate forum for determinations of decisional capacity. The norms of hospital practice, however, do not lead in that direction, and there is a general societal acceptance that in most cases, patients, caregivers, and family can more privately, informally, and sensitively reach consensus as to the patient's abilities in a certain circumstance.

Most patients are either clearly capable or clearly incapable of determining what it is that they desire for themselves. If patients consent to a proposed intervention, few would think to challenge their capacity to give such consent. This is probably appropriate if one assumes that most proposed interventions are suggested because they are in the patient's "best medical interest," that is, the medical benefits to be gained from the intervention, either cure or comfort, outweigh the risks of the intervention to the patient.

Since the choices of most people coincide with what is "best" medically for them, it may therefore be in no one's interest to question a patient's capacity when she consents. (Note, however, that such a proposition demands a tremendous amount of trust and faith that caregivers act only out of concern for what is medically best for their patients—a potentially questionable assumption given the competing demands on modern caregivers.)

There is uncertainty, however, about the ability of certain patients to give consent. Such questioning is often prevalent when the patient is elderly.

It is almost always raised when a patient, elderly or otherwise, refuses a proposed therapy or intervention. While it is clearly wrong to declare someone "decisionally incapable" merely because they choose the "wrong" option (i.e., they disagreed with the opinions of caregivers and did not provide the anticipated consent), it would not be wrong for caregivers to probe the patient's reasoning in the context of the refusal. The *outcome* of the patient's selection does not necessarily indicate cognitive deficits or diminished decisional capacity, but studies have documented that patient refusals are often the product of misunderstanding of important information, or miscommunication with caregivers, situations that can be addressed and resolved.

The decisional capacity of certain elderly persons is often, unfortunately, routinely questioned, and theoretically determined, even before such persons are presented with the option of consenting or refusing. In fact, caregiver biases and the fluctuating or compromised cognitive abilities of many elderly patients may lead to the unnecessary and unfortunate removal of the elderly person altogether from the decision-making process. It is often true that the very reasons leading to an acute care hospitalization, and the actual hospital setting itself, lead to fluctuations or diminutions in the elderly person's abilities. Pain and discomfort from the disease process, as well as secondary infections, nutritional deficiencies, or toxic metabolic reactions to prescribed medications, could all significantly affect the patient's decisional capacity at any given point in time. Moreover, the change in setting to the sterile, unfamiliar hospital environment, with its constant flow of strange faces and the restrictive demands of hospital routines, has been documented to lead to confusion and disorientation in certain elderly persons. The question for caregivers to address is whether such periods of confusion or fluctuating capacity necessarily mean that the elderly patient is unable to make individually appropriate choices regarding her health care.

Most scholars (though perhaps fewer clinicians) have come to view capacity as not only specific to the context and factors of the decision in question but "time" specific as well. That is, persons who have fluctuating periods of capacity or confusion should be consulted and questioned during those moments or that "window" of lucidity comes, when they are better able to focus on the factors necessary to make the decision. For example, it may be appropriate to discuss proposed interventions with an elderly person early in the day, before fatigue and other factors compromise abilities. In turn, it may be necessary to await the resolution of a fever before the patient achieves enough clarity to contemplate her options. Certain emergency situations may not permit this sensitive and perhaps time-consuming search for decisional capacity, but it is imperative that those who care for the elderly accustom themselves to the different time table that may be necessary in caring for, and treating, the elderly patient. Such sensitivity is crucial if the elderly person is to retain her fundamental rights and role in the process of decision making directed toward her health care.

What about the elderly patient, however, who lies in the shades of gray—that is, the patient who has no clearly discernible moments of lucidity, who has permanent cognitive deficits or perhaps memory losses consistent with the onset of dementia? How should caregivers determine if such a person can reasonably, much less legally, give an informed consent or refusal? Unfortunately there is no one clearly articulated legal standard to which caregivers can readily turn. However, based on an amalgam of case law, scholarly works, and standards articulated by a presidential commission convened to examine legal and ethical issues in the delivery of health care, the following factors can be put forth as relevant to determinations of decisional capacity: (1) The presence of evidence that on some basic level the patient comprehends such relevant facts as her current situation, the expected prognosis, the options available to her, the risks and benefits of the proposed intervention, and, in particular, the consequences to her of whatever choice she articulates for herself. No one demands or expects a patient to possess sophistication or expertise equal to that of a physician in matters regarding health care. Yet in order to feel comfortable that they are not abandoning a truly incapacitated patient, caregivers must in some way sense a basic level of comprehension from the patient.

(2) The patient should possess a set of values, preferences, or moral/religious beliefs. Patients may not be able to recite a consciously thought out or cogently articulated set of principles that guide all of their actions, but on some level they may be influenced by an unspoken set of preferences or priorities, so that their presently articulated choice seems to "make sense" given the course of their lives. For example, such concerns as independence, privacy, or esthetic pleasure may be of the utmost importance to a certain individual, such that she would rather die than risk being permanently tethered to a machine, or she would rahter succumb to the ravages of cancer than lose a limb or a breast. A more concrete example is the person of Jehovah's Witness faith who would prefer the risk of death than to be damned in the hereafter because of a blood transfusion. An elderly person, having lived a long life, may possess deeply felt and fundamental, albeit idiosyncratic, beliefs. Others may disagree with these concerns or may not prioritize them in quite the same way, but a caregiver's knowledge of individual preferences may help to explain and support the choices of an elderly person. In such circumstances, close family members or friends may play a crucial role in validating the "authenticity" of the patient's choice, i.e., confirming whether such a choice is consistent with prior actions or behaviors of the patient. The more authentic and consistent the patient's choice, the less likely it is that caregivers will seek to discredit and disempower the elderly person in the decision-making process.

(3) The elderly person must be able to appreciate the complexity of the decision in question and the risks of the proposed intervention: certain scholars have argued that different decisions demand different levels of capacity. For example, choosing among the options available on a hospital breakfast menu requires minimal levels of capacity. If caregivers were wrong in their assessment that the patient was decisionally capable, the worst damage that could befall the patient is a breakfast she wouldn't enjoy. In such a case, the choices are relatively simple and the risks to the patient are minimal. That same patient, however, may not be considered decisionally capable of providing consent or refusal for a proposed quadruple bypass surgery. The complex factors involved in assessing risks and benefits for such an operation, and the potential risks to the patient emanating from such surgery, may place this decision beyond the abilities of the specific patient. Capacity is therefore measured on a sliding scale: the more complex and risky the procedure, the more "capacity" we demand from the patient. Such a construct of capacity is consistent with the notion that capacity is specific to the decision at hand.

It is noteworthy that the above outlined guidelines and factors are somewhat vague and open to interpretation. That is no accident, for the concept of decisional capacity represents evolving opinions, conflicts, and uncertainty in society as to who should be empowered to take what risks in what circumstances. It is a concept of empowerment that straddles our societal notions of respect for autonomy and self-determination on one side and our concern to protect and provide for those truly unable to care for themselves.

INFORMED CONSENT AND REFUSAL

The previous descriptions and discussions of competency and decisional capacity form an important backdrop to the analysis of the consent process for health care decisions. A certain level of capacity is necessary before an elderly patient can decide whether to either consent or refuse a proposed health care intervention. But why is there such concern over this consent process? What does it mean when we say informed consent has been obtained from the patient? What information must a caregiver provide to a patient before such consent has been obtained? What value is to be given to the patient's refusal? Finally, how are decisions made for patients who are too incapacitated to give consent? Are others empowered to decide on the patient's behalf? Such an array of questions demands a thorough examination of the principles behind, and the structure of, the informed consent process.

Bioethical principles and a longstanding tradition in American law have strongly supported the notion that as self-determining, autonomous individuals, patients have the right to decide what health care interventions are personally appropriate for them. Adults in our society are empowered with the fundamental right to control what happens to their bodies. This concept was elegantly and forcefully underscored at the beginning of this century by New York Justice Benjamin Cardozo, who stated, "Every human being of adult years and sound mind has the right to determine what shall be done with his own body."

In more recent years, this common law notion of self-determination has been joined by a constitutionally based "right of privacy." That is to say, in the last two decades or so, a series of U.S. Supreme Court decisions have described and delineated a constitutional right of privacy that has been said to support and shield from public scrutiny or intervention private and intimate decisions about one's body. Thus, decisions to purchase and use contraception, or to obtain an abortion, have been held to be protected under the constitutional right of privacy. This right of privacy has been expanded by several state courts and scholars, to include under its aegis the right to decline life-sustaining treatment. The right of privacy is now generally accepted as one of the fundamental concepts supporting the right of patients to make decisions for themselves.

The philosophical notion of self-determination in the health care setting was originally embodied in the law under the tort doctrine of "battery." Medicine was viewed by the law as a "touching" between provider and patient. In those instances when physicians did not receive their patient's permission, this nonconsensual touching could leave the physician liable for monetary damages resulting from the commission of a "battery." There was, however, no accompanying obligation that physicians inform their patients about the details of the proposed touching. All that was required was the permission itself.

The notion that the caregiver not only had to obtain the patient's permission but had to provide information to the patient prior to accepting such consent is a relatively recent development in the law. As available treatment options began to multiply both in number and complexity, and as the attendant risks to such options became more clear, there came a recognition in the law that the right to self-determination meant little without the concomitant provision of information necessary for a thoughtful consideration of what was being proposed. Thus the obligation for physicians to obtain "informed" consent was born. Those physicians who failed to provide the relevant details of the proposed intervention could now be potentially liable under the legal rubric of "malpractice." Their behavior would be examined as to whether it was so negligent that it fell below the accepted standard of care for physicians. Such liability, however, is contingent not only upon the failure to inform but also on the consequent harm to the patient because of that failure.

Today, when providers or patients think about giving "informed consent," they may conjure up notions of signing a consent form. Such a form is often required for the legal purpose of documenting the patient's consent, but it has little to do with the actual *process of informing* that should take place between providers and patients prior to the initiation of any intervention. Caregivers have the obligation to *talk* with their patients so that the latter can integrate the details of their medical conditions with their value preferences and ultimately reach a personally appropriate calculus of acceptable benefits, burdens, and comfortable health care interventions. Such discussions must occur in a language, and at a pace, that is accessible and understandable to the patient involved—a particularly important point for the caregivers of the elderly to remember.

The specific details of what must be presented to the patient vary depending upon the state in which the patient resides (medical malpractice standards are the product of state laws and regulations as opposed to *federal* law determinations). Certain states mandate that physicians must meet the "reasonable patient" standard: they must disclose all details that a "reasonable person" in the patient's position would consider material to making the decision. Other states, however, have a "reasonable physician" standard, which requires the physician to disclose to the patient all information that a "reasonable physician" in circumstances similar to that specific physician would disclose to a patient. The "reasonable physician" standard is the more commonly accepted standard.

Whichever standard is applicable, there exists a general consensus that certain key pieces of information should always be shared with the patient. These elements include the following: the patient's diagnosis, prognosis, a description of the proposed intervention, its risks and benefits, and the existence of alternative options and their risks and benefits. These are all factors considered fundamental to the patient's ability to render an informed opinion as to the proposed intervention. An unfortunate but common practice among some caregivers is not to include elderly persons in the decision-making process at all, or to turn to relatives for the required consent. This is, however, ethically and legally impermissible, so long as the patient has sufficient capacity to make a decision. Advanced age in and of itself should in no way disqualify a person from rendering an informed consent or refusal.

There are, however, certain legally recognized, albeit limited, circumstances under which the normal process of informed consent is suspended. Such exceptions will generally fall into three categories: (1) The emergency situation, when to obtain consent is either impossible or would cause injurious delays; the law *presumes* consent on the part of the patient. The assumption is that most people would want to be attended to under emergency conditions. This "presumed consent" is most operable and present in hospital emergency rooms. However, once the crisis has resolved, the caregiver would have the obligation to seek the patient's consent, if possible, should further interventions be warranted. (2) The "therapeutic privilege" for certain *limited* circumstances in which the law permits caregivers to refrain from seeking the patient's consent if the physician has a reasonable and well-founded belief that the process of informing itself would be so psychologically harmful or distressing to the patient as to cause significant injury or harm. Caregivers must be careful, however, not to permit this exception to swallow the rule of informed consent: presumptions that the patient "could not handle the information" more often reflect caregiver discomfort regarding the potential discussion rather than concrete evidence that the patient is too psychologically fragile to discuss her situation. (3) Circumstances under which the patient herself chooses not to participate: At certain times a patient may clearly "waive" her right to give informed consent. She may feel more comfortable delegating that right to decide to another, perhaps to a close family member or even to the involved physician. Such delegations are permissible but unusual, such that a caregiver should not presume such a waiver is in existence without some prior explicit statement from the patient.

Case law and bioethical theory not only support the right of the capable patient to give informed consent but just as strongly support the coequal right of the capable patient to give an *informed* refusal. Adult patients with decisional capacity are permitted to refuse a proposed intervention, even if the consequence of such a refusal could be serious injury or death. If the right to self-determination is to mean anything, clearly it should support an elderly person in her decision not to allow someone to touch her body or tamper with her systems, if that is not intervention she desires. The patient's refusals, however, should result from the same knowledge and thoughtful reflection that consents represent.

There are certain interests recognized by society that at times may stand in opposition to the patient's right to refuse, particularly if the refusal could lead to the patient's death. On rare occasions, one of these interests may even override the respect normally given to such refusals. These recognized interests include the sanctity of human life, the protection of third parties who are dependent on the patient, the societal desire to prevent suicide, and finally the need to protect the integrity of the health care professions.

While the law recognizes the dignity of all human life and the need to protect innocent third parties, these two interests have rarely been held to outweigh the right of a capable, autonomous person to decide what is best for herself. Most often in such cases, courts of law are concerned about minor children who may be left orphaned because of their parent's refusal of treatment. Such concerns would be rare with regard to elderly patients.

Judges and philosophical scholars have clearly and consistently distinguished a patient's refusal of a proposed medical treatment from a person's consideration of, or attempt to commit, suicide. Allowing a disease process to take its course is morally distinguishable from the intentional self-termination of an otherwise "viable" life. Physicians who respect the refusals of their patients are in no way viewed as "assisting a suicide" (which is an action still potentially susceptible to criminal prosecution in certain jurisdictions).

While there is clear societal recognition of the role of health care providers to help cure and rehabilitate their patients, there is also a shared understanding that caregivers should comfort their patients and ease the pain and suffering of those under their care. Being a good provider does not always mean *doing* something "for" (or more likely "to") the patient. It may also mean comforting and supporting a patient who decides she has gone through enough, a patient who wants no more intervention. It may be that the personal values of an individual caregiver are such that the individual feels uncomfortable with, or unable to respect, the patient's preferences. That is an understandable situation, and in most cases a physician or other caregiver may be able to withdraw from a case, provided the patient is not abandoned and suitable alternative arrangements are made. In very few circumstances, however, is the need to preserve the integrity of the medical profession so weighty as to override the capable patient's choice to refuse unwanted treatment.

Whether a patient decides to either consent to or refuse a proposed treatment, it is clear that a patient must possess a certain level of decision-making capacity. What is also required, however, is an atmosphere conducive to making a thoughtful, informed decision: in particular, an atmosphere free of pressure or coercion (perhaps a difficult demand in an era of cost containment and efficiency endeavors). The concept of self-determination not only implies the need for knowledge, it also calls forth the notion of freely made, voluntary decisions. An individual can hardly be considered autonomous if her decisions are made under duress or are forced upon her.

The requirement of voluntariness in no way implies that caregivers should not express their opinions as to what they consider to be in the patient's best medical interest. Patients look to their caregivers for advice and consultation. It is up to the caregiver to convey her expertise and judgment honestly. However, in matters of values and personal, religious, or moral preferences, health care providers have no particular expertise or special training. They must be sensitive to separate out expert advice and opinion from biased or idiosyncratic judgments as to "right" and "wrong" in a given situation. Consent that is either coerced or fraudulently obtained would be considered legally void and would certainly stand counter to the prevailing ethical consensus that capable patients are owed the same freedom and respect due to all autonomous, self-determining individuals.

In the real world of health care delivery, many forces may stand allied against patient autonomy and voluntary decision making, particularly for elderly patients. The status of being sick, by itself, often leaves the patient in a vulnerable and dependent position. Moreover, providers are trained (and health care institutions are designed) to take control of the situation and to put the patient on the road to recovery. Those patients who opt for a detour may find little support or assistance. Taking a stand counter to what is expected is a true act of courage in the health care arena, especially for a frail elderly person who may be dependent on family, intimidated by younger professional caregivers, and held hostage to the unfamiliar routines of institutional settings. Responsible caregivers should be especially sensitive and attuned to the support elderly patients may require for their personal choices.

PROXY DECISIONS

As previously described, determinations of decisional capacity represent a balance of respect and preservation of autonomy with protection for those patients truly unable to make decisions for themselves. While it is important to enhance and support the self-determination of persons who are capable of making personal choices, it is equally important to recognize the needs, and to prevent the abandonment, of those who are truly dependent. Health care professionals, particularly those in a geriatric practice, will inevitably come to care for a certain group of patients who, for reasons ranging from memory impairment to permanent vegetative state (with all ranges of dementia in between), can no longer select among personally appropriate options. Several issues thus arise for caregivers: Who is empowered to make decisions on behalf of such patients? Family? Friends? Physicians? On what basis should these "substitute" decision makers come to decide? What if the patient had previously expressed her wishes? And what about those patients who failed to discuss issues of care in advance of their incapacity, or who never possessed the capability to consider their options? The answers to all of these questions are found under the realm of what the law and bioethics describe as "surrogate" or "proxy" decision making.

In the general course of affairs, adult individuals expect to be able to make decisions for themselves and to transact their personal affairs without assistance. Under certain circumstances, however, this may not be possible, either because of physical incapacity, illness, or perhaps because circumstances necessitate an absence from home for a period of time. In such instances, there is availability of a legal mechanism whereby one adult individual formally and legally empowers another adult individual to be his legal "agent" or "proxy." This arrangement is known as a "power of attorney."

Powers of attorney originally became popular in this country to meet the financial needs of soldiers away from home. While a soldier was away, he needed someone to handle his banking transactions and other financial matters. Thus the power of attorney relationship was invoked: One capable adult, known as a "principal," would formally empower another capable adult, known as a "proxy," "agent," or "attorney-in-fact," to legally transact business and conduct other determined affairs on behalf of the principal. According to the law, then, the proxy, whose scope of enpowerment is set by the principal, acts however the principal would act and behaves in the same legally binding manner in which the principal would behave.

The principal has the right to make this relationship with the proxy as expanded or limited as she pleases: the proxy may be able to handle all the business affairs of the principal, or his access may be limited to certain select bank accounts or other financial endeavors. It is up to the principal to define the scope of the empowerment. As well, the principal can hand over to the proxy what is known as a "durable power of attorney." The term "durable" means that this legal relationship survives and continues beyond any mental incapacity the principal may experience. A regular power of attorney is only valid so long as the principal remains mentally intact. That is because the proxy is only empowered to transact those affairs that the principal himself could transact at that specific time. By declaring the power of attorney "durable," however, the principal ensures that the proxy will remain empowered despite any incapacity that may befall the principal. Such an arrangement is quite logical given that it is precisely at the point of the principal's incapacity that proxy decision making would most likely be required. Under either the regular or durable power of attorney, the proxy's empowerment ends immediately upon the death of the principal. Conversely a capable principal can revoke and rescind the proxy's empowerment whenever he so chooses.

Powers of attorney are most often used in the context of financial dealings, particularly for access to bank accounts or stock transactions. The question that many state legislatures have addressed, and many caregivers have considered, is whether such formal fiduciary relationships of surrogate decision making could be employed in the context of health care decisions. While it is thought that general power-of-attorney laws would be available for those sorts of decisions, many states have enacted new legislation that explicitly and specifically permits the use of durable powers of attorney for health care decisions. Under such arrangements, the principal, in advance of any future illness or incapacity that may set in, legally empowers the proxy to make whatever health care decisions are necessary for the sake of the principal, if at some future time the principal herself does not possess decisional capacity. Ideally, the principal, prior to empowering the proxy, should have serious and thoughtful discussions with the proxy, so that the proxy will be well aware of, and will be able to act upon, the personal preferences and desires of the principal regarding potential health care interventions.

Caregivers and patients can call upon either their local bar associations, or local medical societies, to determine the exact availability of these types of legal arrangements in their own communities. Different states have different requirements regarding such issues as the documentation necessary for a durable power of attorney arrangement, the limits imposed on the proxy's empowerment, and the conditions necessary in order for the power of attorney mechanism to be invoked. In most cases, the assistance of an attorney is not required to arrange for a power of attorney, although legal consultation may be advisable in more complex situations.

Usually, a notary is required to witness the principal's signature on the power of attorney form. In all states, the power of attorney relationship ends upon the death of the principal. Such an arrangement has no connection with such matters beyond the principal's death as the handling of the principal's will or estate, or the method of payment for the funeral arrangements.

As the above description implies, proxies appointed through power of attorney arrangements may hold a sizable amount of power and discretion over important aspects of the principal's life and well-being. In the law, this arrangement is known as a "fiduciary" relationship, as it is built upon notions of trust, faith, and obligation between the two parties. Obviously the principal must therefore feel comfortable with whomever she is appointing to this powerful position, be it a family member, close friend, or even a trusted caregiver. The principal may choose any one she wants as the proxy, though finding a trustworthy proxy with whom she can feel at ease discussing these issues may not be an easy task. Nonetheless, caregivers should encourage their elderly patients to consider such arrangements, for they help ensure that patients consider issues and preferences well in advance of crisis and that caregivers have a knowledgeable and informed surrogate to help make decisions according to the patient's personal preferences, should the patient lose decisional capacity at some future point.

Despite the benefits to be gained through the use of power of attorney relationships in the health care context, and despite their increasing popularity and acceptance, such mechanisms are not yet routinely employed by geriatric patients and their families. Only a few elderly patients enter the health care arena with court-appointed surrogate decision makers already in place. Even if a patient does have a court-appointed committee, conservator, or guardian, few of these legally appointed guardians will be specifically empowered by the court to make health care decisions for the patient. A conservator or guardian appointed to manage a person's finances may lack the skill, knowledge, or motivation to make personally appropriate health care decisions for the patient (although misunderstanding of the law and common practice probably leads *de facto* to the empowerment of these court-appointed guardians in the health care setting).

If a patient has failed to appoint a proxy in advance, and no court-appointed surrogate is already in place, how are decisions made for a decisionally incapable elderly patient? Should caregivers take it upon themselves to decide for such patients? Should a court-appointed guardian be specifically sought for the particular medical decisions at issue? What about the rights and the role of the family, or of close friends, in the decision-making process?

The normal routines of a health care practice rarely lead to courts of law under such circumstances. For the few incapacitated patients who have no family, or in cases of controversy, when perhaps caregivers and family disagree as to the appropriate course, judicial involvement may be necessary and appropriate. Particularly for those elderly persons who are voiceless because of their incapacity and vulnerable because no family member steps forth as the patient's advocate, a neutral, objective court of law may be the best decision-making forum. After all, the job of the judicial system is to protect the rights of the voiceless and defenseless.

In most instances, however, providers will turn to family members when elderly persons are decisionally incapable. (An unfortunate and *in-appropriate* behavior among some practitioners is to turn to family members directly, even when the elderly patient *is* decisionally capable, thereby violating the right of that patient to make decisions for herself.) Such arrangements usually occur without the benefit of judicial validation. Is it ethically acceptable, much less legally valid, to turn to the next of kin, despite their lack of legal empowerment to make decisions on behalf of their elderly relative?

In terms of legal liability, such a practice is so common and so well recognized that it is highly unlikely (with the possible exception of extremely controversial cases) that any legal sanctions would attach to such arrangements, despite the lack of a formal court appointment. Moreover, case law and statutes in many jurisdictions specifically permit familial decision making in the absence of a formal legal guardian. Such a practice, so routinely employed, is commonly accepted because in most cases, it is the family of a patient, or perhaps a close friend, who knows the patient best and has the patient's best interest in mind. While there are occasional occurrences of family dispute or even a conflict of interest among family members, in the majority of cases caregivers appropriately seek the help, guidance, and input of family members for decisionally incapable patients. In a sense, a close family member is a "natural" surrogate for an incapacitated elderly patient, for such a person, more than any other, may best know the intimate values, desires, and preferences of the patient, and can advocate for these factors in the context of the decision-making process.

Those persons appointed or selected to be a patient's proxy decision maker can find guidance for their task in two different standards, both of which have the support of case law and the bioethics literature. These two standards are known as the "substituted judgment" standard and the "best interest" standard.

Under "substituted judgment" the proxy for the incapacitated patient woud determine the appropriateness of a suggested medical intervention based upon his knowledge, understanding, or interpretation of the desires and values of that patient: the proxy must attempt to make whatever decision that particular patient would have made if she had the capacity to do so. The proxy might find assistance with this task if the patient left behind written evidence of her wishes (perhaps through either execution of a durable power of attorney or a living will*) or if the patient previously held discussions with her family or caregivers about her preferences on such matters. Clear evidence of what the patient would have wanted should determine the nature and extent of potential medical intervention. Without such concrete evidence, however, a proxy might still be able to look to the patient's value system, religious preferences, or even idiosyncratic notions, so that the proxy will consider the same sorts of factors the patient would have in arriving at a decision.

The reason that the substituted judgment standard requires such a complex decision-making endeavor is due to the desire to maintain respect for the patient's right to choose for herself, despite the incapacity that has set in. Notions of privacy and self-determination are not discarded when a patient loses her decisional capacity. Instead, respect and support for these rights become crucially dependent on the proxy decision maker, who exercises these personal rights on the patient's behalf. It is through the acts and advocacy of the proxy that the wishes of the incapacitated patient come to fruition.

---

*An explanation of the Living Will shall follow.

For some incapacitated patients, however, the task of discerning what their personal desires would be is an impossible one. Certain adult patients (for example, the congenitally retarded) never possessed the ability to consider options or express personal preferences. Other patients never had the motivation or took the opportunity to convey to family or others what their choices would be regarding potentially invasive or unwanted medical care. Family or close friends may be at a loss to evaluate what the patient *herself* would have wanted. Still other patients will have no family or friends to provide the sorts of crucial background information necessary for making a substituted judgment. For the patients just described, substituted judgment is not an available standard for surrogate decision making.

Instead, decisions for these incapacitated patients will have to be made according to the "best interest" standard. Such a standard of surrogate decision making shifts the focus of concern away from the subjective and idiosyncratic factors particular to the individual patient. Instead, what becomes important are more objective criteria related to the medical intervention, including the risks and benefits to the patient of the proposed intervention, the patient's potential for pain and suffering, and the success of the potential intervention in light of the patient's underlying prognosis. Since individual values and personal preferences are missing from the decisional grid, decisions are instead made according to what a "reasonable person" would choose under the circumstances. According to legal theory, factors attributable to a "reasonable person" are those commonly accepted and societally shared notions of what a "reasonable" person under similar circumstances would consider.

It is quite possible that a decision made for an incapacitated patient under the "best interest" standard would differ markedly from one made under the "substituted judgment" standard for that same patient. As previously implied, the "substituted judgment" standard is preferable, if the necessary information is available, since it attempts to enhance and support the personal preferences specifically identified with the particular patient at issue and thus respects such fundamental rights as privacy and self-determination. However, if the appropriate, subjective information is lacking for a substituted judgment, then it is thought best to make decisions for the patient based upon objective, medical considerations.

ADVANCE PLANNING

For many elderly persons, their later years can be a source of pleasure and enjoyment. Their time is their own: old hobbies can be renewed with vigor and new interests can be undertaken and explored. Retirement and "the golden years" can be an exciting and fulfilling period in one's life.

Yet a carefree attitude of relaxation and freedom from responsibility is not always the aura that dominates one's later years. For many, there may be fear of the future: what lies ahead is uncertain, though there is the likelihood of some physical decline and the inevitability of death at some future point. A sense of powerlessness to stop the inevitable, and loss of control in the face of deterioration, may overwhelm an elderly individual. An often crucial role of a geriatric caregiver is thus to help an elderly client face her fears and anxiety and to assist the person in her attempts to maintain as much control over her life as is comfortable, and to define the parameters of the future to whatever extent possible. Concrete planning for the future, in terms of the individual's legal, financial, personal, and medical needs, can be a critical way to assist the elderly person in facing the future and maintaining contol over her life.

A difficult but important act in the lives of many elderly persons is the drafting and execution of a will. In general terms, the drawing up of a will is part of an individual's "estate planning": that is, planning for the future distribution and ownership of one's assets and property upon one's death. An individual need not have a will in order to have property distributed to family members upon death. Each state has laws that govern the ownership of assets of persons who die "intestate," i.e., without a will. There is a legally set pattern of distribution of a deceased person's property, depending on the nature and extent of the relatives left behind.

However, an individual may not agree with the mandated pattern of property distribution set by state laws for persons who die intestate. For example, for whatever personal reasons, an individual might want to leave all of her money to one child, rather than having her property equally distributed among her several children, as the state's intestacy laws would require. By drafting and executing a will, then, a person may plan for the future ownership of her property according to whatever idiosyncratic factors she wishes.

Carrying out personal vendettas beyond the grave is not, however, the only reason an elderly individual should be advised to have a will. In fact, a will can be a very personal and positive force in one's life. It is a method of showing one's gratitude to others, and of providing for and protecting family and loved ones. In fact, any individual upon whom others are financially dependent should have a will that arranges for the continuation of this financial arrangement (if that is desirable) upon that person's death. Very often, relationships exist that have no legal foundation or support—it is only the commitment and the existing arrangement that underlies the relationship. Without provisions in a will, such arrangements may disintegrate or fail to survive the legal challenges of others.

Moreover, a will is not only for the purpose of distributing property or allocating financial interests. It can be, as well, a vehicle through which very important and personal statements and desires can be articulated and carried out. For example, an individual may want to express her deep love or affection for some particular person through a will, or she may want to make her personal preferences known regarding funeral services or burial arrangements. Used for these reasons it becomes clear that having a will is not only appropriate for wealthy individuals but for any person with strong concerns or desires about matters that will go on beyond her death. Of equal value are the senses of security, empowerment, and control that accompany the drawing up of a will.

As stated previously, each state has specific laws governing the distribution of assets upon a person's death. Not only do such laws cover circumstances of death for which there is no will but there are particular laws and regulations that outline the procedures and technicalities that must be followed in order for a will to be legally valid and binding. Such laws are often very complex and confusing; consultation with an attorney is strongly recommended to ensure the legal validity and force of whatever terms make up the will.

Despite the different requirements state by state, a few generalizations about the drafting of a will are consistent nationwide. For example, just as with any important decision, when drawing up a will the individual must possess *capacity* and be acting *voluntarily*. Persons declared legally incompetent may not be legally permitted to draw up a will (though a previously existing will, drawn while the person *was* legally competent, would most likely remain valid despite the present declaration of legal incompetency). Even the wills of those persons still presumed legally competent could be subsequently challenged on allegations of incapacity.

In general terms, an individual who is drawing up her will should know the following: (1) she is participating in the drafting of her will; (2) the nature and extent of the property that she plans to distribute; (3) those persons whom the law would consider her "natural" beneficiaries, i.e., close relatives or next of kin; and (4) those persons to whom she is actually distributing her property, and the reasons for doing so. A will may be declared invalid or void if the testator (the person whose will it is) was lacking one of these elements of knowledge while her will was being drawn up. As well, wills drafted under duress or coercion may also be subsequently invalidated. If a will is invalidated by a court, and no previously drafted and valid will exists, then the property will be distributed in accord with the state intestacy laws.

If they have not previously done so, elderly persons may want to consider and utilize other mechanisms of estate planning. For example, to avoid the cost and procedures involved in drafting and probating a will (that is, having the terms of the will carried through under court supervision), an elderly individual may want to give all or partial ownership of her property to another prior to her death. A common and often very useful endeavor for an elderly person is to arrange for bank accounts, for example, to be held in joint ownership with another, often an adult child. The account would be set up under terms "with a right of survivorship," such that once the elderly person died, the account would automatically become the legal property of the other person named on the account, with no need to refer to a will or to have a court intervene. In addition, trust accounts can be arranged that permit the elderly person to control her money while she is alive, but legally and automatically transfer the funds to the named beneficiary upon the elderly person's death, again without the need of a will. Insurance policies with designated beneficiaries work in the same way.

Various tax consequences and other considerations accompany the myriad of options. Local attorneys and financial advisors are best able to counsel the elderly person (even the person with few assets or little property) as to what is most appropriate and advantageous for the particular person's needs and desires. Such planning can also assist the elderly person in maintaining a comfortable and secure lifestyle for the remainder of her life. Caregivers of geriatric patients or clients should have access to local referrals.

The need to plan for the financial future of others or for property distribution upon death may be an individually difficult task, but it is a societally accepted and expected endeavor. While possibly reminding an elderly individual of her own ultimate mortality, such planning may also underscore a sense of security and control: her own future and that of her loved ones has been attended to and she stands as the master of her own property and possessions. It is by her choice and her decisions that others will have to abide. No one questions an individual's decision to document such preferences through the execution of a will.

A less common, but increasingly recognized form of "advance planning" has to do with the documentation of preferences regarding potential health care interventions. The past several decades have been witness to a technological explosion in the health care arena: a variety of chemotherapeutic agents and mechanistic interventions now exist to maintain hearts beating, lungs breathing, and blood flowing well beyond the ability of the brain to maintain sentience or relational capability. To some, these advances represent modern man as scientific genius. To others, this innovation represents technological enslavement, as elderly individuals become tethered to machines and entangled by tubes, all in the name of maintaining life. In fact, the majority of persons in this country now live out their final hours and days within the confines of an acute care hospital, where the use of such technology is a fact of everyday life. The question that many elderly persons now face is whether such a finale is acceptable to them, and if not, how to ensure a less scientific (and perhaps more humanistic) close to their lives.

As noted earlier, elderly persons with decisional capacity possess the clear legal and moral right to consider the range of potential health care interventions that may await them, and to provide their consent or refusal to specific treatment suggestions. While not all scenarios can be planned for or anticipated, individuals can nonetheless contemplate potential and foreseeable circumstances, and can make their desires known accordingly. Consultation with, and the advice of, the elderly individual's primary caregiver is essential for this type of advance planning. It is in fact suggested that caregivers, be they physicians, nurses, social workers, or other trained professionals, have the obligation to initiate such discussions with elderly persons under their care, and to elicit if possible and document the patient's preferences or choices.

Thus, the patient's informed and articulated desires would be available to guide and control the decision-making process, should the patient subsequently become decisionally incapacitated. In this way, elderly persons can ensure that they maintain control over the direction of their lives, and caregivers can avoid the thorny and distressing ethical dilemmas that often arise in the care of elderly, incapacitated patients. At times when proxy decision makers are necessary, such proxies will have the clear and articulated evidence necessary to make a substituted judgment.

Caregivers can document the patient's wishes as part of her medical records, or in the patient's hospital chart. In either the acute care nursing home or the home care setting, all members of the patient's health care team should be informed of any specific desires or choices the patient may have expressed. Caregivers should encourage their elderly patients to share with family members or close friends whatever directions they have given to their caregivers, so that all parties potentially involved in future health care decisions are cognizant of the patient's desires. In fact many elderly persons may look to their families to help them consider and think about such advance plans. It is, however, ultimately the capable patient's choice as to how much information she chooses to share with relatives or friends.

Beyond their documentation in the individual's hospital chart or medical record, the preferences of elderly patients regarding future medical care may also be recorded in specifically drafted documents, known primarily as "advance directives" or "living wills." The majority of states now have "Living Will Legislation" (often called "Natural Death Acts"), which specifically permits and empowers individuals to document their wishes in a specially written form, in case future decisional incapacity leaves them unable to address medical care options. These living wills only become operative if the individual patient is incapacitated at the time the health care decision needs to be made. If drafted under the terms and circumstances defined in the legislation, such living wills would be legally (and morally) binding upon caregivers. Using this planning mechanism, an elderly individual can ensure that caregivers know of and respect her wishes, despite her inability to articulate them.

Even in states that have no specific living will legislation, nothing legally prohibits an elderly person from drawing up a personal document that clearly and explicitly details her wishes in case of future mental incapacity. In fact, geriatric caregivers should work to encourage their capable patients to address and document, by whatever method (i.e., living will, durable power of attorney, or notes in the medical record), their desires regarding the use of such sophisticated machinery as respirators, dialysis, or feeding through nasogastric or gastrostomy tubes. The method of documentation is not nearly as important as the depth of the discussion and the informing of those caregivers and family members who are in a position to act upon the elderly individual's preferences. Given the technological treadmill on which an elderly person may find herself once hospitalized in an acute care facility, the need to consider potential interventions well in advance of need or future incapacity is essential: for patients who wish to maintain control over their lives *and* deaths, and for caregivers, who are often forced to choose between the availability and use of sophisticated machinery on one hand and their respect for patient autonomy and obligation not to cause needless suffering on the other.

DETERMINATIONS OF DEATH AND POST MORTEM ACTS

With an array of technological interventions available to extend lives (and, some may argue, prolong the process of dying), the exact point of death is often a difficult, agonizing, and perplexing determination. This may be particularly so for family members, who may feel the warm touch of their relative's skin, or see the heart of their loved one still beating, perhaps due to the use of a respirator. The machinery exists today to replace the failed major body organs, even if the brain is no longer able to coordinate their running and functioning. In these days of medical advances, the question becomes, what in effect constitutes the death of an individual?

Various religious groups have traditionally demanded the lack of functioning throughout the *entire* body before death could be declared. Some religious individuals, such as followers of Orthodox Judaism, still look to this "heart-lung" standard, believing an individual to be alive until the last breath has come, even if that breath comes as the result of artificial breathing machines. In many jurisdictions, however, the legal definition of death has shifted away from the "heart-lung" standard to a criterion that examines brain stem function. Such a shift has come about due to the excessive use of technology that often maintains organ function well beyond the body's viability, and to the increasing success of organ transplant programs that transfer the organs of newly deceased individuals to the bodies of otherwise dying individuals. Over the years, transplants of kidneys, hearts, and other major organs have saved the lives of innumerable otherwise doomed individuals. The success of these transplants is, however, highly dependent on the retrieval of the organs promptly after brain death is declared. The longer body organs are artifically maintained after brain death, the less viable they will be for transplantation purposes.

Today, a great many states (New York among the most recent) have formally enacted legislation or regulations recognizing brain death as the legal point of death, rather than the absence of circulation or respiration. Under such laws, the total absence of brain function, including brain stem activity, indicates the person's death. Specific medical tests are outlined in the laws to make this determination carefully and with certitude. Many states have an "either/or" policy, such that either brain death or respiratory/circulatory failure constitutes the death of the individual.

Despite the attempts at legal clarity, determinations of death and the consequences that follow (such as the cessation of all medical care and intervention) still remain muddled at times, and often occur under emotionally charged circumstances: religious preferences may not coincide with legal declarations, families may be unable to accept the loss of their loved one, and patients with minimal brain stem activity (with no hope of recovery) lie in a legal limbo, never to regain sentience but nonetheless subject to continuous medical intervention because such individuals cannot be considered legally dead. The heart of this debate often centers on individual notions of the essence of "personhood" as opposed to the mere existence of biological functioning.

What happens to the body of the deceased once there is a clear determination of death may also be problematic. Persons are legally empowered to document wishes with regard to such post-mortem activities as organ donations, autopsies, or funeral arrangements. Theoretically, these documented wishes should then be respected. However, old common law notions about "ownership" of the deceased's dead body by the next of kin and sensitivity to the desires and preferences of the grieving family may prove to override whatever preferences the deceased documented. It is the rare caregiver or hospital official who will override or ignore a family's refusal to consent to autopsy or organ donation, despite wishes of the deceased to the contrary. Therefore, individuals who have strong feelings about these post-mortem activities would be wise to discuss and make known their preferences well in advance of their death, so that calamity and chaos do not overwhelm the already difficult process of dying and death.

THE ELDERLY IN THE POLITICAL ARENA

The statistical data is clear: the size of our population that is sixty-five years old and older is increasing at a faster rate than younger groups and, in particular, the population that is eighty-five years old and older constitutes the fastest growing segment of our entire population. Estimates are that presently, twenty-nine million Americans are over the age of sixty-five, and by the year 2010, that number will climb to thirty-nine million. While most elderly persons are in good health and free of serious illness, the incidence of chronic and acute disease does increase with age, such that concerns about the cost and availability of hospital services, long-term care facilities, hospice programs, home care, community support services, and low cost prescription drug programs are all important central concerns in the lives of elderly individuals.

Coincident with this increasing rate of growth of the elderly population is, not surprisingly, an increase in their political clout. National lawmakers such as the late Congressman Claude Pepper from Florida (who died recently at the age of eighty-seven) are increasingly encountering more receptive audiences with regard to issues of primary concern to the elderly. In fact, older Americans now constitute a dominant force in American politics. This is particularly so given the large voter turnout among older citizens. Statistics from recent Congressional elections highlight this fact: while the elderly represent 16 percent of eligible voters, they accounted for 21 percent of the actual voter turnout in 1986 Congressional elections.

Organizations and lobbying groups devoted to issues affecting the elderly are now considered major players on the American political scene. One of the first elderly activist organizations, the Gray Panthers, has now been joined by a myriad of groups representing various aspects and interests of our geriatric population, including such organizations as the National Council of Senior Citizens, the National Senior Citizens Law Center, the National Citizens' Coalition for Nursing Home Reform, and, most notably, the American Association of Retired Persons (AARP). Considered the most politically powerful and influential voice in American politics regarding issues of aging, AARP has a membership of over twenty-eight million members (eligibility is open to all citizens, fifty years old and above), employs a thousand people as staff members, and runs on an annual budget of over

$190 million. This powerful association has successfully sponsored and supported major political initiatives intended to prevent benefit cutbacks and to expand the available coverage of such benefit programs as Medicare. The support and endorsement by groups like AARP are now political prizes for those seeking elected office.

While efforts are continually underway to devise and develop new publicly funded programs to benefit the increasing geriatric population, an array of well-established entitlement and benefit programs already exists. Some of these programs accrue to the elderly merely because of chronological age; others require income or means tests to determine financial, as well as age eligibility. The following description highlights some of the most prominent national and state programs designed to provide support and benefits to elderly individuals:

Social Security

The United States Social Security Act was passed in 1935, largely in response to a shift from a rural economy, supported by agricultural endeavors, to a more urban economy where income was derived from wages paid through employment arrangements. At that point in our history, political and societal recognition united (spurred on by the Great Depression of 1929–33) about the need to protect and provide security for older workers unable to earn an income due to lost employment opportunities or to the necessity of retirement.

With additional programs and amendments tacked on in the years since 1935, the Social Security Act now supports a variety of financial assistance and support programs to four main groups in our society: the elderly, the blind, the disabled, and dependent children. Of most interest and concern to elderly individuals are those programs encompassing retirement benefits, survivors benefits, disability and health insurance.

Most elderly persons are eligible to receive Social Security either based on their own employment history or that of their spouse's. Individuals who retire at age sixty-five or older become eligible to receive their benefits; those who choose to retire at an earlier age (from 62-64 years) are eligible for their social security benefits at a reduced percentage of what they would have received had they retired at age sixty-five. Persons seventy-two years of age or older are entitled to begin receipt of social security benefits even if they are still employed at that age. The actual amount of the benefit is based upon the average annual taxable income of the previously employed individual. The surviving spouses and dependent children of deceased social security recipients are also eligible to receive a percentage of the entitled worker's benefits.

Beyond retirement benefits, elderly individuals may be eligible for other types of social security payments. For example, the survivors of an insured worker become entitled to one lump-sum payment upon the death of that worker. As well, eligible workers and their dependents may become eligible for Social Security Disability (SSD) payments, depending upon their employment history and the nature and extent of the disability in question. Local Social Security offices should be able to help determine an individual's eligibility for these various programs. Caregivers should have handy reference to such local offices.

Title XVI of the Social Security Act also authorizes a program that assists many elderly persons of more modest or limited means. Known as Supplemental Security Income (SSI), the program provides monthly *income* assistance (as opposed to health care related assistance) to elderly, blind, or disabled individuals. Such disability includes both physical and mental incapacity, determined through a physician assessment. To determine financial eligibility for this program, an individual's income and assets are considered and taken into account.

Medicare

The Medicare program provides health insurance to those sixty-five years of age or older, and to certain disabled individuals below the age of sixty-five. This program was created in 1965, under Title XVIII of the Social Security Act. The idea for a health insurance program of this sort arose at the time the original Social Security Act was being considered, but the actual passage and implementation of the Medicare program only came about with the support of Presidents Kennedy and Johnson.

The Medicare program is composed of two parts, each of which covers separate areas of service delivery. Part A coverage, which comes automatically to all eligible recipients, covers such areas as in-hospital services (exclusive of phone and television service), a very limited amount of nursing home and home care services, and certain hospice services. Part B coverage, which eligible recipients must specifically opt for and for which recipients must pay a small monthly premium, applies to certain physician services, diagnostic tests, medical equipment, and other outpatient services and therapies.

Part A coverage under Medicare provides full reimbursement, after payment of a deductible, for the first sixty days of a patient's hospitalization and partial reimbursement for the days thereafter. This is applicable for each incidence of hospitalization. Additionally, a beneficiary is given a one-time reserve of sixty additional days for illnesses requiring extended hospitalization. (Note, however, that Congress recently passed legislation intended to provide extensive coverage for catastrophic illnesses that necessitate prolonged hospitalization. Caregivers and patients can contact local Medicare offices regarding the details of this newly extended coverage.) Elderly individuals can, in addition, purchase supplemental insurance coverage, available through such groups as Blue Cross or even AARP, for coverage beyond the Medicare reimbursement. Without this supplemental coverage, individuals are personally responsible for bills not covered by Medicare.

The Medicare reimbursement system has gone through a dramatic shift in the past several years. This shift has refocused the reimbursement mechanism for hospitalization away from fees set according to the discretionary services directed by the physician to a payment schedule set by the patient's specific diagnosis. Several hundred Diagnosis Related Groups (DRGs) have been established under the Medicare system such that a specific diagnosis will bring the hospital a fixed payment, regardless of the amount of time a patient spends in the hospital or the amount of intervention necessary to assist the patient in her recovery. It is highly likely, therefore, that hospitals will spend more on the care of certain elderly patients than they will receive in Medicare reimbursement. Too many such patients could cause significant financial problems for acute care institutions.

Given this new payment mechanism, there is continuing concern that elderly patients might be "short changed" on their care, or might be discharged earlier than is medically reasonable, due to the financial pressures on caregivers and hospitals. Caregivers and patients alike should be well aware that Medicare patients have the right to dispute or challenge reimbursement levels or denials. Nonetheless, this unavoidable infusion of financial concerns into the caregiving arena may lead to significant conflicts of interest for caregivers, who pride themselves on being patient advocates yet have responsibilities and loyalties to the institutions with which they are affiliated (as well as concerns about their own income levels).

Medicaid

Medicaid is a program designed to pay for the health care expenses of eligible individuals of limited financial means. Funding for this program comes from both the federal and state levels, and each state has a certain amount of discretion as to which services it will provide under its own Medicaid program. The Medicaid program came about as Title XIX of the Social Security Act in 1965.

Eligibility for Medicaid is determined by examining an individual's level of income and amount of assets. Certain individuals are automatically eligible to receive Medicaid. Such persons are considered "categorically needy," meaning that because they already receive certain types of public assistance, they are automatically entitled to receive Medicaid. Included among such individuals are those receiving SSI (described above) under the Social Security system, and those receiving AFDC (Aid to Families with Dependent Children). Additionally, in many states, persons who are considered "medically needy" may become eligible to receive Medicaid. Such individuals usually have incomes or assets slightly higher than is permissible under Medicaid regulations, and they become eligible for Medicaid by "spending down" their excess income or assets on their own health-related expenditures. Local Medicaid offices can provide caregivers and patients with the details regarding such "spend down" options.

Many elderly individuals, having exhausted their savings on their medical care, ultimately become impoverished to the point of becoming Medicaid eligible. This is particularly true for residents of nursing homes, where the high cost of institutionalized care virtually wipes out within a matter of months the savings of all who enter such facilities. Medicaid, in fact, provides more funding for nursing home care than does any other source of reimbursement.

Eligibility for Medicaid can be a complex and complicated determination for an elderly person, particularly if both spouses are still living and their finances are joined. Different states have different eligibility requirements, but states are permitted to consider the assets and income of one spouse as available to pay for the cost of the other spouse. Such considerations are called "deeming." In the past, such deeming practices have led to the impoverishment of a spouse in the community when the other spouse has had to be institutionalized. Advocates for the elderly are now fighting such dire consequences, and in New York there are court cases that have permitted spouses to refuse to contribute toward the other spouse's institutionalization and even allow the community spouse to sue the institutionalized spouse for support payments, so that the community spouse is not forced to spend her remaining days alone and impoverished. There are attorneys and financial planners now available to help elderly persons protect themselves from impoverishment while becoming Medicaid eligible. Caregivers would be wise to have reference to local reliable professionals who can provide this type of financial planning and advice.

The services provided through Medicaid reimbursement vary from state to state, though a range of inpatient hospital services, nursing home services, and physician services are provided in every state. While Medicaid recipients are generally free to choose whichever caregiver they want, the state-set reimbursement levels to caregivers accepting Medicaid patients are often quite low, such that many caregivers refuse to take on Medicaid patients. In many areas, therefore, the actual care available to Medicaid recipients is quite limited.

Beyond these well-established federal and state financed programs, an array of additional services and other spending policies exist for the benefit of elderly persons. In fact, the federal government now spends, in total, about 20 percent more on the elderly than it does on our nation's defense. Much of this funding is distributed to local Area Agencies on Aging (AAA), which are organizations that receive federal monies through the Older Americans Act. With more than 600 such agencies in existence nationwide, a variety of social and health-related services are made available to persons sixty years old and older.

For example, specific food, nutrition, and housing programs exist to benefit elderly persons. Such programs are designed to meet the basic nutritional or housing needs of elderly persons of modest means, or those who may be home-bound due to incapacity or chronic illnesses. Included among these services are programs such as the Food Stamp Program (jointly administered by federal and state agencies) or local "Meals on Wheels" programs. The "Meals on Wheels" programs are usually administered by AAAs, which provide home-delivered meals (usually one meal per day, five days a week) for a small fee to homebound elderly persons. The AAAs may also provide low-cost meals to senior citizens through local community or senior centers. Some communities even sponsor home-delivered meals to the elderly on weekends as well.

In addition to nutritional concerns, housing-related problems are usually another major source of concern for elderly individuals. Such concerns may range from the care and upkeep of long-held property to decisions to move to alternative housing arrangements, including "senior homes" or skilled nursing facilities (often called "SNFs" or more commonly, nursing homes). Many elderly homeowners are entitled to reduced property or income taxes. Often low-income elderly persons can receive help for winter fuel bills. Those seniors on fixed incomes may in fact qualify for certain reduced cost, governmentally financed housing programs. In certain communities, housing has been constructed specifically for elderly persons, often with rents well below market price. Other housing programs provide rent subsidies to qualified elderly individuals. Local senior citizen groups are likely sources of information on these housing-related programs for the elderly.

While consideration of, or entrance into, a nursing home may seem far removed from the purview of the public or political arena, in fact, most nursing homes are subject to federal and state regulations designed to assure a minimum quality of care, and to support and define the rights of residents living in such institutions. Such regulations oversee policies relating to admission, transference, treatment decisions, personal activities, and financial transactions. Under mandate from the Older American Act, every state must have a long-term care "ombudsman," whose specific job it is to investigate and resolve the complaints of nursing home residents in that state.

Beyond the traditional "board and care" homes or nursing homes available to dependent or incapacitated elderly persons, an increasing variety of alternative options is developing for elderly persons no longer willing or able to maintain their long standing places of residence. For example, local senior organizations have been instrumental in developing shared housing programs, which may provide companionship, cost-saving, and maintenance free living in the community for elderly persons who might otherwise be forced to enter institutional settings. A specific type of shared housing arrangement known as "congregate housing" is available in some communities. In congregate housing environments, special services are available for the elderly resident, including transportation, meal preparation, and housekeeping services. Usually residents will have individual apartments but communal meals and activities will be available. As with other types of elderly service programs, local offices on aging are probably best equipped to describe to caregivers and their elderly patients the options available in a specific community.

FUTURE POLITICAL ISSUES CONCERNING THE ELDERLY

Despite the rather impressive array of services, benefits, and entitlement programs already available for elderly persons, several major areas of concern are likely to appear on the political agenda in the near future. Foremost among these issues will be financing for long-term care of the elderly. This is simply because Medicare provides virtually no reimbursement for long-term care, and Medicaid coverage is only available to those elderly individuals impoverished because of their high medical expenses. At present, private, affordable insurance coverage to meet circumstances necessitating long-term care is scarce. Thus, elderly persons not only face the fear of physical and mental incapacity caused by long-term chronic illnesses but they also must worry about their ability to pay for care and to attend to their basic needs and comfort, or they must bear the emotional pain caused by the need to call on their children or other relatives for support. Proposals to expand Medicare coverage for nursing home or homecare services have begun to surface. Yet a national consensus has yet to be achieved in this important area.

As voices continue to cry for additional spending programs for the elderly, an increasing concern has to do with the basic question of justice and the appropriate allocation of increasingly scarce resources in this country. Given that 30 percent of the federal budget is already allocated for programs for the elderly, and that this group accounts for only 12 percent of the population at present, there is the danger of a backlash against older people who, by and large, are better off than other age groups in society.

Intergenerational competition may force us as a society to question and rethink why we treat the elderly as we do. Already, major writers from the areas of philosophy and social policy have begun to raise the unmentionable, i.e., rationing based on age, particularly regarding the availability of expensive, high-tech medical care. Other countries, such as Great Britain, have openly and frankly faced those issues in public. In this country fear of political backlash and genuine uncertainty about our notions of justice and equity have prevented overt policy making. Instead, allocational determinations become the *de facto* consequence of the large, impersonal, and at times ill-conceived bureaucratic decision making.

The upcoming explosive growth of our elderly population will force this country, however reluctantly, to consider and come to terms with our societal obligations to older persons. Careful, concerned, and sensitive debate will have to address such issues as the privileges that should accrue to the elderly *merely* because of chronological age, the obligations society can legally and morally impose between and among familial members (particularly between adult children and their elderly parents), and the appropriate allocation of increasingly limited resources, particularly in an era of increasing poverty among children and increasing prosperity among the elderly. Despite the fear and concern that the specter of such debate may raise for certain individuals, it is necessary that we, as a society, address these issues and that we do so in an open, public, and intellectually honest way. The consequences of such debate may not be comfortable for all, but the process of reaching such decisions must be accountable and inclusive, so that all those affected, particularly the elderly, may be guaranteed that their concerns will merit serious consideration and attention in the decision-making process. If one thing is clear, it is that we owe the elderly no less than this inclusion and concern.

FOR DISCUSSION

1. Determinations of decisional capacity seem to balance the desire to respect the patient's status as that of an autonomous, self-determining individual with concerns about the patient's safety and risk. Describe what factors are crucial to this determination, particularly for a frail, elderly patient.
2. When is it appropriate to involve family members in the health care decision-making process for elderly patients? If an elderly patient refuses to consent to this familial participation, what, then, are the obligations of the patient's caregivers?

3. What types of issues or interventions should a patient address in her Living Will? Should caregivers encourage all of their patients to make such advance plans or just those patients who are already ill? Which individuals should have knowledge of, or even a copy of, a patient's Living Will?

4. What reasons can be put forth to justify special treatment of the elderly by the government, in terms of benefit availability, taxation rates or budget allocations? Should elderly persons be entitled to differential treatment merely because they are elderly or should they be required to show financial need as well? Are any other groups in society entitled to these kinds of special privileges?

REFERENCES

American Association of Retired Persons, *The Right Place at the Right Time: A Guide to Long-Term Care for the Elderly.* Washington, D.C.: A Publication of Health Advocacy Services, Program Department, American Association of Retired Persons (1985).

American Hospital Association, "A Patient's Bill of Rights." (1972.)

Annas, George J., *The Rights of Hospitalized Patients,* an American Civil Liberties Union Handbook. New York: Discus Books, Avon Press, 1975.

Butler, R. N., *Why Survive? Being Old In America.* New York: Harper & Row, 1975.

Kapp, M. R. and Bigot, A., *Geriatrics and the Law.* New York: Springer Publishing, 1985.

Kapp, M. R., Pies, H. E., and Doudera, E. A., *Legal and Ethical Aspects of Health Care for the Elderly.* Ann Arbor, Mich.: Health Administration Press, 1985.

Office of Technology Assessment, Congress of the United States, *Life-Sustaining Technology and the Elderly.* Washington, D.C.: US Government Printing Office, OTA-BA-306 (1987).

President's Commission for the Study of Ethical Problems in Medicine and Biomedical and Behavioral Research, *Deciding to Forego Life-Sustaining Treatment.* Washington, D.C.: U.S. Government Printing Office, 1983.

President's Commission for the Study of Ethical Problems in Medicine and Biomedical and Behavioral Research, *Making Health Care Decisions: Volume One.* Washington, D.C.: U.S. Government Printing Office, 1982.

Regan, John J., *Tax, Estate and Financial Planning For The Elderly*. New York: Matthew Bender & Co., Inc., 1985.

Robertson, John A., *The Rights of the Critically Ill,* an American Civil Liberties Union Handbook. Cambridge, Mass.: Ballinger Publishing Company, 1983.

10

Ethical Concerns

Connie Zuckerman

INTRODUCTION

Ours is a time of both expansion and decline in terms of America's elderly population, and each of these directional trends highlights positive and negative aspects of growing old in contemporary society. Expansion is clearly the trend when examining the sheer size and numbers of our geriatric population. Accompanying this explosive demographic data are concomitant increases in the available opportunities and technologies that permit our elderly citizens to lead more comfortable, productive, and meaningful lives. On the negative side, however, this same population expansion signals an unfortunate increase in the number of individuals who suffer from chronic disabling illnesses and conditions. These people are in need of increased social support and health care services.

Decline has become an important term, especially regarding the elderly. The decline in mortality rates clearly illustrates the longer lives our citizens are leading. The same term is often used to describe the physical and cognitive functioning of older persons. For most elderly persons, their advanced years bear witness to declining abilities, frequently in terms of physical capacity and often in terms of mental agility as well. Today's elderly (along with the rest of society) are quickly facing another aspect of decline, one that we have struggled to fend off and ignore: the decline of resources available to meet *all* of their possible or potential needs (particularly regarding health care). We have tried to deny that the pie is limited, but reality seems to tell us otherwise.

The most vivid illustrations of the issues just noted are to be found in current demographic data and the predictions they engender. Current figures and estimates appear to support some eye-opening assertions. While the elderly (those sixty-five and beyond) constituted 11.3 percent of the American population in 1980, this proportion is expected to expand to 13.1 percent by the year 2000, and increase to 21.7 percent by the middle of the twenty-first century. In more concrete terms, the population explosion of elderly persons is expected to be the prime reason for increases in the following by the year 2050: the number of annual physician visits (up 47 percent); the number of short stay hospital days (a 100 percent increase); the number of persons needing assistance with such basic daily activities as eating, walking, and personal hygiene (up 152 percent); and finally, the number of persons occupying a nursing home bed (the figure will jump by 246 percent). Those dramatic figures can be coupled with a projected drop in the proportion of the population of twenty- to sixty-four year olds from 58 percent in 1982 to 55 percent in 2050.

Countless dilemmas and conflicts become self-evident once these trends and figures are pondered: Are we to applaud this exponential growth of our elderly population? Is a longer life necessarily more valuable or fulfilling? Does this growth necessitate that we draw or define limits regarding societal obligations to meet the increasing care needs of our elderly population? Must we more sharply determine the nature and extent of the obligations, duties, and responsibilities between and among family members, particulatly adult children and their elderly parents? What principles or policies shall we use if in fact we must begin to ration, or more restrictively allocate, scarce resources? How will we know whether our actions are "right" or "wrong"? Will it become necessary to examine more consciously the *quality* of life, and not merely its extension? Who will define and decide what is a worthy, valuable, and "supportable" quality of life (in terms of the expenditure of public funds)? What part will (and should) the elderly themselves play in these emerging national debates? And what about the elderly who possess diminished mental abilities? How can we (and should we) consider their preferences and desires?

These are but a few of the many troubling and perhaps tragic conflicts we are likely to face. They raise questions about the very core of life and its meaning, and about the fundamental structure and vision of our society. As one prominent scholar has posed the issue,

> The way a society treats its elder members depends to a large degree on the value it attributes to old age. The value of old age to a society depends in turn upon its views about the meaning or purpose of life. And a society's views about the meaning or purpose of life are formulated

primarily to help make sense out of the inevitability of death. Thus it is apparent that in any given society there is a close connection between its treatment of the elderly and its philosophy of death and dying. [Edmund Burke, "Death and Aging in Technopolis: Towards a Role Definition of Wisdom," *The Journal of Value Inquiry* 10 (Fall, 1976)]

One could argue, then, that our present societal ambivalence about the role of the elderly, the value of their lives, and the obligations of society and the family to support their growing needs is merely a reflection of our ambivalence and discomfort with our inevitable mortality. Nonetheless, the coming explosion in the geriatric population demands of us that we openly, honestly, and equitably address many of the concerns raised above, for the betterment of both our present elderly citizens and for the future members of this expanding population.

ETHICAL PRINCIPLES AND ANALYSES

Before we can substantively examine many of the questions just raised, a brief digression is necessary to outline the function and major principles of our ethical analyses, particularly as they apply to this examination of the elderly.

Some may wonder of what use is a discussion of philosophical principles or abstract notions about moral obligations; after all, we have laws in our society that define for us acceptable and unacceptable behavior. Such a limited vision, however, ignores the fact that in a heterogeneous society, the system and substance of our laws reflect both politically-engineered compromises on broad notions of morality and also the means by which we ensure a minimum degree of social control. As such, there are many aspects of individual behavior that remain ungoverned (and ungovernable) by legal structures. These are often areas of behavior too intimate or morally problematic to ever succumb to regulation by judicial determinations or legislation. This is particularly so given the need for laws to be practically enforceable in addition to politically palatable.

There are also technological advances, particularly in the health care context, that outpace existing laws or, in turn, bring to our attention conditions not previously considered ripe or appropriate for legal intervention. In sum, gaps are left that the law cannot, or does not yet, address and thus the need for ethical analyses becomes apparent. Such analyses can provide us with the values and spirit that should influence, if not direct, our behavior, either in the absence of existing laws or even in their presence. For it is clear that what laws define as acceptable may not, in fact, coincide with an individual's notion of what is in essence the morally appropriate action in a given circumstance. (In fact, the very consideration of civil disobedience or violation of the law demands that we account for and prioritize our own moral values and guiding ethical principles.) Thus, in either the absence of law (as a precursor to future law) or even as an alternative to existing law, ethical analyses can help define for us both the options available, and the principles of consideration, in situations of ambivalence or unclarity.

In the area of bioethics (the application of ethical theories and principles to the practice of medicine and biomedical research) four major principles (put forth by Beauchamp and Childress) are generally agreed upon as fundamental to the evaluation of behavior in terms of its "rightness" and "wrongness." These principles are particularly germane to our investigation of the elderly, their desires and needs, and the possible just limitations on the fulfillment of those needs, particularly in the health care setting.

Principle of Autonomy

In both bioethics and case law, the principle that adult individuals should be self-determining, i.e., free to decide what is right for themselves according to personal schemas of morality and individual value preferences, is a fundamental concept. In terms of health care, this principle of autonomy means that adult patients have the right to make personally appropriate decisions about their health care and about proposed medical or surgical interventions, i.e., they have the right to give informed consent or informed refusal. Having provided patients with the appropriate information, caregivers grant patients the dignity and respect they are owed as autonomous individuals by respecting whatever informed decision the patient reaches. One should note, however, the ongoing dispute over what level of functioning a patient should demonstrate before her choices are considered the product of an autonomous, self-determining will and thus worthy of respect. In contrast to the positive rights of patients, the picture of autonomy has a negative dimension, i.e., it is a shield preventing unwanted intrusions. What remains unsettled, however, is whether a *positive* notion of autonomy is equally legitimate, i.e., whether positive claims for access to care or specific interventions are equally deserving of recognition and respect.

The Principles of Nonmaleficence and Beneficence

The second major principle is that of nonmaleficence: the proverbial "do no harm," to which physicians and other caregivers pledge themselves upon entrance into their professions. Such a principle requires that caregivers neither injure their patients nor inflict harm upon them by either negligent or intentional act. This is not so much a positive claim for action on the part of caregivers as it is a negative call of forbearance, a prohibition on harmful conduct. This principle of nonmaleficence is often coupled with the third principle, that of beneficence. In contrast to nonmaleficence, beneficence does in fact require positive action on the part of caregivers, not the merely abstaining from negative or injurious conduct. Beneficence includes within its meaning both the positive obligation to prevent or remove harm and the duty to promote the patient's welfare or provide a benefit. When in a position to do so, caregivers have the positive duty to act beneficently, and to contribute to or enhance their patient's well being.

The Principle of Justice

The final principle is that of justice, an important one in the examination of the place of the elderly in our society. In general terms, this principle has to do with the recognition of what is due or owed to an individual, either because of some inherent moral properties she possesses or because of her status in relation to other individuals or groups. Individuals can demand that they be treated justly when they make claims for what they rightly deserve. In contrast to justice on the individual level, there also exists the broader concept of *distributive justice,* which has to do with the distribution of both benefits and burdens across members of society. In times when resources are scarce and competition keen among those who claim these resources, a principle of distributive justice helps define the most equitable and just method of allocating such resources.

On many levels, a just method of allocating increasingly scarce health resources has yet to be worked out in our country. Thus, individual caregivers are often left in the awkward and unfair position of choosing between competing claims, perhaps resulting in unfair consequences or acts of discrimination against certain patient populations. Elderly persons, who are often frail, nonaggressive, or unable to advocate on their own behalf, may be at particular risk for being treated unfairly when resources are scarce and societal consensus has yet to be achieved on acceable allocation principles.

The concepts briefly outlined above are by no means exhaustive in terms of the scope of circumstances they cover. They constitute, nonetheless, basic principles that enjoy general support from the two major strands of philosophical debate that dominate the field of bioethics: (1) the *consequentialist* tradition, which defines the moral "rightness" of actions on the basis of the *consequences* of those actions, with particular attention given to those consequences that produce the most benefit to the greatest number of people, and (2) the *deontological* tradition, which defines a series of duties or obligations incumbent upon individuals regardless of their consequences, in order for their actions to be within the orbit of morally acceptable behavior. In the discussion that follows, it will be evident how even the most concerned and sensitive of caregivers, whatever her philosophical bent, may nonetheless encounter distressing conflicts and competition among these four principles, particularly when it comes to the delivery of health care to elderly individuals.

AUTONOMY VERSUS BENEFICENCE
IN THE CARE OF THE ELDERLY

The philosopher Immanuel Kant (1724–1804), whose theories of duty and respect for persons have had an enormous impact on the field of bioethics, described the inherent moral dignity that lies in each of us because of our unique ability to make rational choices. It is this ability to reason that permits us to act autonomously, according to Kant, and grants us our status as autonomous beings who demand respect from those with whom we interact. As autonomous individuals, we should always be empowered to determine what is best for ourselves.

To act as an autonomous, rational individual in the context of health care decisions would mean, ideally, that the patient would come to make a personally appropriate decision ofter the caregiver has carefully laid out the patient's options and explained the choices. However, the perfection envisioned in the Kantian world is rarely glimpsed in the often impersonal and imposing real-world settings of acute care hospitals or long-term care facilities. Circumstances of the setting and the practice of medicine tend to work against the smooth application of Kantian notions of autonomy. Moreover, patients may at times exhibit behaviors or articulate choices that could lead caregivers to question the person's *capacity* to act autonomously (a topic left unaddressed by Kant). Other perceived caregiver obligations toward patients, beyond respecting abstract notions of patient autonomy, may complicate the caregiver's agenda, Kantian wisdom notwithstanding.

Particularly with regard to elderly patients, there is often the question (be it founded or unfounded) as to whether the patient has the requisite mental capacity to *permit* her to act autonomously or whether, due to diminished capacity, the patient needs more protective intervention on the part of the caregiver. A clear corollary to the obligation to respect the autonomous decisions of patients is the need to protect the well-being of patients who, because of diminished capacity, are unable to promote their own welfare or best interests. The obligation to act beneficently may loom just as large in the caregiver's mind as the obligation to respect the patient's autonomy.

The focal points of this dilemma concern the definitions of the concepts of capacity and autonomy, terms not synonymous but often interrelated when it comes to examining these sorts of decisions. Conflict may occur when a patient's expressed desires regarding medical treatment or intervention seemingly lead her down a path that is inconsistent with what *others* perceive as being in the patient's "best interest." Determinations then need to be made as to whether the patient's expressed desires or "spoken choices" truly reflect an "autonomous" decision or, rather, some other incapacitating condition, such that the patient does not possess the ability to be autonomous ("self-ruling") at least in terms of this decision.

What it means for a patient to be acting "autonomously" is still a debatable concept for philosophers and others interested in this more esoteric aspect of patient care and behavior. It is, by and large, settled in the literature and the law that if a patient is considered to be making an autonomous decision, then that choice necessitates respect from caregivers regardless of the fact that this choice conflicts with the values or judgments of others about what is appropriate for the patient. But what does it mean to say that the patient is acting "autonomously" so that caregivers must abide by her wishes, even if idiosyncratic or bizarre?

One particularly thoughtful scholar, Bruce Miller, has outlined four different senses of the concept of autonomy, at least as it is used among medical ethicists. First, according to Miller, there is the sense of autonomy as "free action" such that the patient's choice is arrived at in an intentional and voluntary manner. For example, an elderly patient who gives informed consent (or refuses to give consent) to have a simple diagnostic procedure performed on her could be considered to be acting "autonomously" if her choice was made without duress or coercion, and if it were her deliberate objective to submit to such a procedure (or refuse to submit). This is a relatively simple and clear notion of autonomy, though perhaps some would claim not "weighty" or thoughtful enough to universally command respect.

Next, Miller shifts to a slightly different notion of autonomy, that is, one that reflects the concept of "authenticity." Here he means that the patient's spoken choices "make sense" in terms of that person: the patient is acting "in character" or in continuation of a pattern of preferences, likes, desires, etc., that she has previously exhibited. There is a consistency or predictability in this person's actions such that if a specifically articulated choice is not in the patient's "best interest" it may nonetheless deserve respect because it is an authentic expression in terms of this patient's value scheme.

Miller then elaborates a more sophisticated notion of autonomy, that which he calls "effective deliberation." Essentially, this category encapsulates the commonly accepted understanding of what it means to give informed consent. That is, when confronted with a situation requiring a decision, a patient would consider her choices, evaluate the consequences of those options, and arrive at a decision after considered deliberation. Such a sense of autonomy incorporates a deliberative process of decision making, in contrast to the previously described senses of autonomy that outline more impulsive, less reflective assertions of choice.

Miller's final category of autonomy is described as "moral reflection." This concept of autonomy requires of an individual the most demanding levels of inquiry. It includes deliberation, as previously described, but also acceptance and utilization of a set of moral values throughout the process. Choosing from among particular options would not only entail consideration of details specific to those options but it would also include a broader reflection on (and at times reconsideration of) the personal values that underlie the choices one makes.

If somewhat complex, these various concepts of autonomy nonetheless demonstrate that "respecting the patient's autonomy" is in fact no easy matter. Whether one chooses to honor the articulated desires of an elderly patient may, then, turn on what sense of autonomy the caregiver considers appropriate to the situation and probably, what consequences may lie ahead if in fact the patient's choice is respected. For example, consider an elderly diabetic patient, admitted to the hospital for a gangrenous condition in her leg. When her physician begins to inform her about the need for surgery in order to halt the spread of infection, the patient refuses to continue the discussion. She simply states, "No surgery," and asks that she be discharged to go home. According to Miller's description of the various senses of autonomy, we might conclude that this patient's refusal represented "free action" in that without coercion or duress she made her choice. It was her intent to refuse the surgery. We might also consider her action "authentic" if we knew, for example, that throughout her life this woman always refused medical intervention, because she preferred to accept whatever fate brought her way. She may have even been brought to the hospital involuntarily. Under these conditions her decision could be termed "autonomous" and thus deserving of respect.

Yet, having refused to engage in a discussion with the physician, much less be informed as to the potential options available to her, it is unlikely that this patient engaged in the type of "effective deliberation" envisioned by Miller. Given the potential ramifications of this refusal, including a slow and painful death as a result of gangrene, it would be reasonable to argue that a caregiver would be obliged to assist this patient in considering all of the options before accepting a final decision. Lacking that deliberation, one *could* argue that this patient's refusal is not fully "autonomous" and that declining to respect it might well be justified. In fact, given the physician's concurrent obligation to act beneficently and to promote the patient's well-being, one might even suggest that the caregiver *must* override the patient's choice, particularly in light of its possible consequences and the less than full sense of autonomy it represents. With elderly patients this dilemma is often further complicated by the additional concern that the patient does not even *possess* the capacity to deliberate effectively about the choices.

Individuals generally make choices and arrive at decisions that in fact do promote their own well-being, as defined by themselves and their caregivers. In such circumstances, there is no conflict between the caregiver's obligations to both respect patient choice and promote patient well-being. These obligations only come in conflict when the articulated choice of the patient appears contrary to, rather than in furtherance of, the patient's well-being (at least as defined by the caregiver). Such a clash is possible when the patient determines that other concerns are more important than what is considered, strictly speaking, in her "best medical interest." For example, the patient may conclude that preservation of a certain lifestyle or quality of living should take precedence over a certain level of health or functioning. In what may ultimately be, then, a clash of *values* between patient and caregivers, there is no "right" or "wrong" answer, such that a caregiver would normally be obliged to put aside personal values as the price for respect of patient autonomy.

Yet another possibility exists as to why the patient's articulated choice may not coincide with what is generally viewed as in her "best medical interest." Various patients, including certain elderly patients, may suffer from conditions that render them mentally incapacitated, such that they no longer possess the ability to even consider or promote their own well-being, however they might have envisioned it within their own personal value schema. Merely being disoriented to time or place, or having short-term memory problems (as many elderly persons do) would not necessarily put someone in this category. Significant impairment in cognitive functioning or the presence of a major psychiatric disorder, however, may render the patient unable to determine what is best for herself—unable, perhaps, to even come to a decision that Miller would label as "authentic." In such cases of "diminished autonomy," it would do violence to the notion of respect for autonomy to accept the patient's choice, particularly if its consequences could lead to serious risk or harm to the patient. Respect for such a "nonautonomous" decision would be tantamount to abandoning the patient: respecting the choice of such an incapacitated person cannot constitute respect for autonomy or for the person in general. Under such circumstances, the obligation to act beneficently would guide caregiver behavior.

Some theorists would term this intervention into the lives of incapacitated patients "justified paternalism." That is to say, the intervention would be considered "paternalistic" in that it was prompted by concerns rooted in the welfare or well-being of the patient, and "justified" because the patient's incapacity leaves her in need of such protection or intervention. Such an act of paternalism stands in contrast to other sorts of interventions that in fact lead to the disempowerment or denial of autonomy for patients who are perfectly capable of making decisions for themselves. For example, caregivers may at times withhold certain information from patients; worse still, they may deceive their patients in order to achieve a desired result. The classic case is that of a caregiver not wanting to reveal all of the risks of a proposed treatment because of concern that the patient will ultimately refuse the treatment if informed of the risks. In essence, the caregiver has determined, according to her own values, that it is in the patient's best interest to undergo the treatment despite the risks and without referral to the patient's personal notions of acceptable versus unacceptable risk. Such interference with the patient's right to make an informed decision would, in most circumstances, be ethically unacceptable despite its appeal to what is considered "good" for the patient. The danger with such paternalistic notions is that they tend to dismiss genuine disagreement over values (about which reasonable people may disagree) as cases of patient incapacity, thus justifying the intervention. Caregivers of the elderly need to be particularly mindful of unjustified paternalism based on a dismissal of the patient's own values.

TREATMENT DECISIONS IN THE FACE OF DEATH AND DYING

Perhaps nowhere in the context of medical decision making is the issue of patient autonomy and control over the decision-making process more important than in the realm of dying and death. Coming to terms with mortality is an inevitable issue that the elderly, perhaps more than other patient group, will face. Historically, it is a topic that caregivers have inadequately discussed with their patients. Disease and death are the ultimate enemies for many caregivers. Recognition of death's inevitability may signal defeat for the caregiver, both in terms of patient well-being and in terms of professional satisfaction. Nonetheless, dying and death are as much a part of human life as birth and maturity. Caregivers often assist patients in recognizing and adjusting to various stages during their lives. It can be argued that these professionals have an obligation to help patients live with and adjust to circumstances in their final days of life.

Many caregivers have argued that, in fact, patients cannot handle such discussions and, in their wake, would lose confidence or the will to live, both of which are considered important psychological components for continued existence. Nonetheless, national surveys continually dispel these myths: patients have generally expressed a wish to be informed of their diagnosis, however dismal, despite physician discomfort regarding the disclosure of such information. There may, in fact, be some tact and sensitivity necessary in planning the form and content of such discussions, but this is not to suggest that they should not be held. For the most part, caregivers have the moral obligation to make available to the patient the option of such a discussion. This is particularly so given the array of sophisticated yet potentially burdensome medical interventions often available to extend or prolong an otherwise failing life.

In fact, it is owing to the development of technological methods to mechanically assist, if not replace, a variety of body functions that many of these dilemmas about death and dying have arisen. For example, beginning in the 1940s and carrying through to developments in the 1960s, procedures were developed to restore heart beat and heart rhythm in patients who experienced a cardiac arrest. Once the technology became available, it was soon commonplace for hospitals to develop emergency resuscitation teams whose members could immediately respond in emergency cases of cardiac or pulmonary arrest (an incident known in medical parlance as calling a "code"). But having the technology available and outlining what *can* be done in a certain circumstance, leaves unanswered the more pertinent question, viz., what *should* be done in such circumstances? This question was asked more often and with increasing intensity when it became "ordinary" for hospitals to subject every patient, no matter what his condition or prognosis, to a code in circumstances of an arrest. This rote application of such a sophisticated procedure often led to devastating results. Patients would "survive" codes only to be left in permanent vegetative states, dependent on mechanical ventilators to support their breathing. What was even worse, patients whose death was imminent and who would experience several arrests in the process of dying, would be continually resuscitated to match these arrests, only to die a painful tortuous death filled with repeated chest poundings and often fractured ribs. The "quality" of death became as much an issue as the quality of the patient's life.

Beginning in the 1970s, many individual hospitals, and later many professional organizations, began to address this dilemma of "automatic" resuscitations. It became clear to substantial numbers of concerned clinicians that a patient's resuscitation status needed to be addressed *in advance* of a cardiac arrest so that sound, rational, and humane decisions could be made in the glare of crisis and chaos. Such "advance planning" would require patient participation or at least familial participation for incapacitated patients. This came in recognition of the fact that decisions to resuscitate a patient or orders *not* to resuscitate a patient (often called "DNR" orders) involved the weighing or assessing of certain risks in the light of certain possible benefits, and the values of the patient were an important component to the calculus of these risks and benefits. Particularly with the potential outcome for the patient of a life sustained by artificial ventilation, it became clear that, if at all possible, the patient had to be a part of the decision-making process. In 1988, in fact, the state of New York actually implemented legislation designed specifically to empower patients and their families in the context of resuscitation decisions.

Other sophisticated technologies include but are not limited to those available in modern-day acute intensive care units. Such individual innovations as artificial nutrition through nasogastric feedings, a gastrostomy tube, or total parenteral (nonoral) nutrition, all raise similar questions about when, given the failure of bodily functions, is it appropriate to offer patients artificial methods to continue body maintenance. Is it always mandatory that all potential options be made available to every patient? Who is to decide both what is offered to the patient and what in fact the patient should receive? Is it ethically permissible for patients to refuse interventions that could prolong their lives? When, if ever, would such refusals be considered suicide?

All of these weighty questions are worthy of in-depth philosophical analysis not possible here. But some brief concepts can be outlined to help students sort through these difficult dilemmas. First, many caregivers mistakingly cling to the belief that morally relevant distinctions can be drawn between the withholding of certain life-prolonging interventions versus the withdrawal of such interventions once initiated. In fact, philosophically speaking, no moral distinction can be made between stopping treatment and not starting it. In the clinical setting, some caregivers may believe that once having started an intervention, its withdrawal for morally sound reasons would somehow implicate the caregiver as an "active" participant in, or cause of, the patient's death. However, a presidential commission that considered this issue in some detail stated, "whatever considerations justify not starting should justify not stopping as well." Moreover, this sort of thinking may precisely work to the detriment of patients, as caregivers may be reluctant to initiate potentially beneficial interventions if they fear that once initiated, they will forever be locked into that course.

Another distinction often made (and one with perhaps more moral grounding) is that between "killing" the patient and "letting the patient die." What is most often thought of in terms of "killing" is the active and intentional bringing about of the patient's death, either at the patient's request or involuntarily. The classic example of this is the purposeful injection of a lethal dosage of narcotics for the *express purpose* of bringing about the patient's death. While the usual intent of this act of euthanasia is the bringing about of a merciful end to a patient's suffering, such active measures are nonetheless commonly considered to violate basic ethical traditions in this country, and they are certainly considered impermissible by law. Direct active killing of innocent persons is generally considered an intrinsic moral wrong. Some argue that in certain extreme cases of unendurable pain and suffering, such active measures may in fact not be wrong. However, exceptions to this general prohibition could lead to a slippery slope: If such "mercy killing" were permitted the acts of euthanasia would not stop there but extend to the active killing of such "undesirables" as the demented elderly or defective newborns; furthermore, the loss of integrity of the medical profession and the loss of patient trust in caregivers would be significant. Whatever the validity of these arguments (and the philosophical debate will continue), it is highly unlikely that active measures to end even the most suffering of lives will be legally sanctioned in the foreseeable future.

Alternatively, the concept of "letting the patient die" has more common acceptance among clinicians and scholars, and it is viewed mostly in the context of permitting patients to refuse life-prolonging interventions. It is not so much that the patient then has a *right* to die (from which some might infer that the patient then has the right to request that someone purposefully assist him in ending his life). Rather, it is that the patient has a fundamental right to be free from unwanted interventions. This is so even if the consequences of such a refusal could lead to the patient's death. As such, the intent of those who choose nonintervention is *not* the express purpose of bringing about the patient's death. This may be a foreseen, but not a primarily intended side effect of the action. Instead, it is to protect the patient's right to bodily integrity and self-determination that such wishes are generally followed.

Hard and fast distinctions between "active" killing and "passive" letting die will sometimes be difficult to draw, and will continue to arouse heated debate in medical and philosophical circles. Take, for example, the disconnection of a patient's respirator after the patient asks for the withdrawal, knowing that he cannot live without such support. While one can clearly argue that the intent of the disconnection would be to respect the patient's choice, nonetheless, the *act* of disconnection will actively lead to the patient's death. Such a case points out the difficulty of using such words as "active" and "passive" as shorthand for much more broad and complex concepts. Nonetheless, clear cases of active, intentional killing, albeit for merciful reasons, will undoubtedly continue to be prohibited in our society, these more subtle distinctions notwithstanding.

Finally, the phrases "ordinary treatment" versus "extraordinary" or "heroic" treatment have been frequently raised in clinical settings in an attempt to distinguish which interventions might be considered more obligatory to offer or accept versus those that might be considered more optional. The origins of this distinction arise from Catholic theology, which used such distinctions to determine the appropriate level of sanction to attach to certain actions; i.e., refusing, withholding, or withdrawing "ordinary" treatments was unacceptable to the church, while actions involving "extraordinary" treatments were more permissible.

In today's sophisticated world of modern medicine, the use of the terms "ordinary" and "extraordinary" probably provides little clarity and much confusion, as these phrases only take on true meaning in relative contexts: that is, what one clinician—perhaps a subspecialist in a large, urban teaching hospital—may consider an ordinary, customary, or commonplace intervention may be viewed as quite rare, unusual, or extraordinary in a different setting—perhaps by a general internist in a rural community hospital.

Moreover, it is quite possible to view the same sort of intervention as "ordinary" in one circumstance, yet "extraordinary" in another, though both may occur in the same setting. For example, it is possible to consider the extensive chemotherapy used in treating the early stages of certain types of leukemia as "ordinary" in that, though inconvenient and the cause of certain unpleasant side effects such as nausea or hair loss, these chemical agents nonetheless have great potential for success and the benefits to be gained by the patient (i.e., remission if not cure) appear to outweigh the short-term side effects or burdens of the intervention. However, the utilization of equally strong chemotherapeutic agents in an elderly person with terminal, metastatic cancer might instead be viewed as "extraordinary," if their use is unlikely to bring about a remission and will lead to a terribly uncomfortable or unpleasant quality of life in a person with little life remaining.

In a sense, then, it is hard to label one specific intervention as either "ordinary" or "extraordinary" unless the intervention is given a context in which such factors can be determined: e.g., its efficacy under the specific circumstances, its benefits in proportion to its burdens for that particular patient, its level of invasiveness, its cost, etc. It is thus easy to understand why abstract categorizations of interventions provide little substantive support in concrete cases. Moreover, even placing the interventions in a specific context will not permit us to attach these labels unless we determine the individual patient's perspective on such issues. If the recognition of patient values in the decision-making process is to mean anything, then it should be the choice of the capable patient to determine what is a personally appropriate balance of benefits versus burdens. An acceptable evaluation of the probabilities of success might help the patient consider one intervention "ordinary" and therefore "acceptable" while another may be "extraordinary" and thus "unacceptable." The problem of personal, even idiosyncratic interpretations and intended meanings is highlighted in the dilemma found in many current Living Wills, in which the patient will claim to refuse "heroic" measures yet leave uninterpreted for his survivors precisely what he considers "heroic." If such vague language is used and subjective interpretation necessary, then it is arguable that the Living Will fails as an expression of the patient's self-determined wishes.

The last distinction that needs a brief examination is that of the issue of suicide and its relationship to a patient's refusal of life-saving or life-prolonging interventions. Most commonly accepted religious traditions in this country strongly condemn the notion of the active and intentional self-induced termination of an individual's life, and Anglo-American law has consistently reflected these traditions. Suicide and the assistance by another in a suicide were not only morally unacceptable but legally prohibited as well. Today, however, most legal sanctions only attach to those who assist in, rather than actually commit, or attempt to commit, suicide.

What needs to be distinguished, however, in the context of life-prolonging medical care, are the origins of suicidal intent. There are those stemming from psychiatric disturbance or mental illness, which are not the consequence of any sort of reasoned or rational considerations but rather the product of conditions that impair judgment and for which psychiatric intervention may lead to a change in attitude. Alternatively, many philosophical traditions argue that, in fact, a supportive case can be made for "rational" suicide, i.e., an individual's decision to terminate his life based on a reasonable evaluation of a present poor quality of life and a dismal prognosis for the future, perhaps because of terminal illness. Individual determinations that such dire circumstances render death preferable to the existing poor quality of life could lead an individual in several directions: the active and intentional suicide, refusal to permit any additional life-extending interventions, or a request for the withdrawal of presently instituted interventions that are maintaining life. Which, if any, of these paths is morally acceptable would depend on the moral schema to which the individual subscribes: certain traditions, while prohibiting the outright and intentional termination of life, nonetheless would find morally permissible actions that permit "nature to take its course." Some moral theorists have even argued that there is no substantive moral distinction to be made among any of the possible alternatives listed above: for them, the most humane, rational, and perhaps cost-effective choice would be to end agony and suffering quickly and actively.

While there may be much legitimacy to arguments pointing to the lack of morally relevant distinctions among these alternatives, the law clearly delineates a path and supports and prohibits certain actions for different reasons. There is in our system of laws a clear philosophical bent toward preserving life: prohibitions on homicide obviously demonstrate this, as do continued penalties for assisting in suicide. Nonetheless, in the context of health care delivery, an equally strong recognition has emerged: that of the right of patients to be free of nonconsensual or undesired intervention, which at times may lead to the inevitable result that a patient dies sooner than he or she might have if the intervention had been undertaken. The law has chosen not to label such refusals as suicide and has consistently upheld the right of capable patients to refuse life-prolonging intervention, despite society's strong notions about the need to preserve life. With less unanimity, and some ambiguity, courts have at times permitted proxies to make such decisions on behalf of incapacitated patients.

Some may point to an inconsistency, if not irrationality, between what is legally permitted and legally prohibited. Certainly, philosophical arguments can be mounted on both sides. But for the present time, suicide remains socially unacceptable while individually motivated actions to refuse life-prolonging interventions continue to gather legal support.

THE ALLOCATION OF RESOURCES
AND THE OBLIGATIONS OF OTHERS

Several years back, the issues of dying, death, and the elderly took on a new dimension, at least in terms of coverage by the popular press. While advocates of the "right to die" and "death with dignity" movements had gained strength and notice for well over a decade, a new debate was sparked when the former governor of Colorado, Richard Lamm, was reported to have suggested that elderly persons not only have a right to die, but in fact they also have a *duty* to do so; i.e., they have an obligation not to use up precious resources that would otherwise be available to younger populations. In a sense, he suggested, the elderly should realize when enough is enough. Such comments provoked a brief but vociferous outcry: such an idea was unheard of, and moreover, unacceptable in a country such as ours. While the public outrage that followed the governor's comments subsided shortly thereafter, the legitimate issue of how increasingly scarce resources should be distributed over a range of needy populations continues to be of concern.

The origins of this debate were sparked, at least in part, by a now familiar theme: the ever increasing geriatric population in this country. Along these lines a few comments must be made. First, out of all health care dollars spent, a disproportionately large amount is devoted to the last six months in the lives of elderly persons, i.e., the dying elderly. Next, the proportion of health care resources devoted to the elderly has gradually and steadily increased, particularly when compared to expenditures devoted to children (some have even argued that this comes at the *expense* of children's needs). Finally, it appears that research efforts and technology aimed at conditions and illnesses of the elderly are eclipsing (and possibly short-changing) the time and efforts devoted by the health care industry to other population groups. In effect, staving off the inevitable effects of the aging process has become a major *goal* of modern medicine, only to be further fueled as the geriatric population continues to grow.

The well-respected philosopher Daniel Callahan, who has been concerned about these issues, recently published a controversial volume aimed at addressing this question of allocation. Specifically, what Callahan suggests in his book is the development of a heightened sensitivity and a new system to address the problem of the vast expenditures to *extend* the lives of the elderly, often with little regard to the *quality* of the life extended. Callahan argues that we are teetering on the brink of financial calamity if we continue to spend large sums on health care for the elderly without, however, truly serving the well-being or the best interests of our geriatric population in the course of these expenditures. Callahan outlines a system of allocation designed to halt the exponential growth of health care expenditures on the elderly while remaining sensitive to the issues of their pain and suffering. Beyond a certain age (which Callahan describes as the "natural life span") the only expenditures permitted on the elderly would be toward the maintenance of comfort, or relief of suffering, as opposed to "valiant" efforts designed to extend or prolong life. In a sense, he suggests a shift from quantity to quality. Callahan proposed such limits in terms of the *public* health care dollars devoted to the elderly are concerned, i.e., through such systems as the Medicare system.

Dr. Callahan's concepts have ignited the public debate as to the most appropriate method for allocating increasingly stretched and ultimately scarce resources. While he gives considerable thought to the development of a humane and just system, it is, nonetheless, a system that ultimately looks to *age* as the trigger for resource restrictions. Many critics find this unacceptable. While Callahan targets his restrictions to precisely the group where there has been the most growth, other theorists argue that less targeted, more neutral principles of resource allocation are the only morally acceptable mechanisms for this unpleasant but ultimately necessary task.

As mentioned early in this chapter, principles concerned with appropriate methods of resource allocation are known as principles of "distributive justice." The issue to be examined, then, is this: given the fact that there are simply not enough "goods" for everyone to always enjoy the most comfortable, happy, and pleasurable life experiences, what is the best method (i.e., the most *fair* method) of distributing benefits and burdens across society? Some needs will have to go unmet. But what principles or criteria are we to use to determine whose needs will go unanswered?

As with other issues of morality, this one has no single right or wrong answer, and it is an issue of continual debate. For example, some theorists espouse principles that look to "neutral" distributive systems. In a sense, no characteristic distinction is drawn between the competing candidates for the limited goods. Allocation is determined simply by such random methods as a lottery system or, alternatively, by such objective considerations as timing, i.e., whoever shows up first at the doorstep of the intensive care unit is admitted, no matter what age, prognosis, or life situation. While perhaps laudable if somewhat idealistic, such a neutral system is rarely utilized in modern health care settings. In fact, acute care facilities often attempt to operate on a "triage" system, at least in emergency settings. Such a system, while not as neutral as the other systems described above, nonetheless attempts to categorize candidates according to the more objective criteria of "greatest medical need" such that those with the most acute, life-threatening conditions are often placed at the top of lists, with therefore greater access to available resources.

Since aging is often accompanied by increased morbidity and the increased incidence of acute events, a triage system might naturally devote disproportionate resources to the elderly population. There are many theorists, however, who attack this sort of objective system. They suggest, instead, that there are legitimate, "subjective" considerations worthy of attention when considering how to allocate scarce resources. For example, it has been suggested that characteristics such as the individual's contribution to society (either past or projected into the future) be taken into account. Perhaps more resources should be available for those who "add the most" to our society. Alternatively, it has been suggested that such factors as patient age, prognosis, "quality of life" or origins of illness (for example, lung cancer attributable to smoking versus another type of cancer not "self-induced") be used to determine who should have access to what resources. Even cost has been mentioned as a possible segregating factor, i.e., procedures beyond a certain dollar amount would not be available (except, perhaps, to the most wealthy who could afford to pay privately).

All of these factors have their advocates and critics. There are philosophical concepts available to support each type of consideration. For example, a consequentialist or utilitarian would support an allocation principle or a specific "subjective" factor if its use would bring about the greatest benefit to the most people, even though a certain minority group may suffer for the benefit of the majority. In turn, individuals with a more egalitarian perspective will only support allocation systems in which all persons will at least have equal access, if not equal care.

As a society, we have yet to take on in any sort of pragmatic, realistic way both the *need* to consider allocation principles and the *actual principles* that should influence policy. That is not to imply, however, that shortages are not now in existence or that mechanisms have not been devised (often on an *ad hoc* basis) to determine who will get access to what types of medical care. In this less formalized, more subtle method of allocating scarce resources, morally suspect and discriminatory practices are more likely to occur, and the elderly are at risk of being excluded from care. In fact, there are many clinicians and scholars who argue that the problem with elderly patients is not too *much* intervention, or the need to be left alone, but rather too *little* care and the need to get more access to certain types of care from which they are being excluded merely because of age alone, or because of others' evaluations about quality of life. This is debatable, but what is clear, however, is that an unfortunate number of individual clinicians have been forced by systemic pressures to confront and act upon what we, as a society, have been too timid to address. In particular, the caregivers of the elderly, squeezed by rigid insurance mechanisms and other regulatory constraints, have been unfairly saddled with decisions and choices about resource allocation, with the unfortunate result, at times, of distinctions being made about who shall live and who shall die.

The squeeze on resources and the availability of support for geriatric patients raises one more issue worthy of brief attention: that of the ability of others, most notably family members, to provide fiscal, physical, or emotional support to their elderly relatives. In particular, as a society, we are just beginning to come to examine this issue of the moral responsibility between and among elderly parents and their adult children. The question is, what, if any, obligations exist for adult children to provide support and care to their aging parents? If such obligations do exist, are they merely supportable by moral imperatives or should we more firmly impose and support such responsibility through legal mechanisms?

In other, less advanced times, familial responsibility and caring for the elderly was a rare and mostly limited obligation. Few people lived to advanced old age and those who did often took on a revered and honored status. It was a blessing to have an elderly relative, as few families could in fact claim that event. Moreover, family systems and structures were quite different. Large, even extended families routinely lived in one household or within short geographic distances. Being a "responsible" relative did not, to a great extent, require the same level of commitment or self-sacrifice that it might demand today. One need only examine the often long distances between today's close family members, and the increased levels of responsibility, including children and careers of their own, for the children (particularly the females) of today's elderly persons.

Moreover, the "burden" of caring for today's elderly parents (as it is often, unfortunately, looked upon) is to a certain extent, the consequence or the "trappings" of our successes as a technologically sophisticated society. To begin with, it is harder, in general, even for the healthy elderly to cope in our society, given the level of technological capability necessary to navigate one's way through the system successfully. The elderly of yesteryear did not have to contend with the frustratingly complex Medicare reimbursement system or with the perils and pitfalls of sophisticated urban living. The type of skills demanded of today's citizens (including the elderly) were not necessary a century ago. Moreover, for those of less fortunate health care status, the equipment and mechanisms needed to maintain their more fragile lives were not available to the elderly and their families years ago. It was simply not an option for an elderly person or her family to have to learn how to handle a colostomy bag or to keep track of complicated medication regimens. In fact, some of our "victories" over disease and illness might be thought of as "Pyrrhic": their costs in terms of the stress and the obligation imposed on both the patient and the family may be too high a price in light of the benefits gained.

In the midst of such a sophisticated society, then, what are the appropriate levels of action and responsibility to demand of the relatives of aging persons? The data from the field of home health care supports the view that, in fact, family members do support and assist their elderly relatives. The majority of home care in this country is provided by "informal" caregivers, i.e., family members (albeit usually the female members). But because family members *are* providing support, this does not necessarily lead to the conclusion that they *should* be providing such support or that such support should be mandated through any sort of fiscal or regulatory public policies. Many elderly persons, in fact, cannot look to family for support, often because no family member is available, able, or willing to meet the needs of an aging relative. Under such circumstances, social or political policy mandating familial support in certain circumstances might unfairly disadvantage those who are, perhaps, the most in need of support and assistance.

Laws that have tried to mandate financial support of elderly parents by adult children have, by and large, been unpopular and unsuccessful in addressing the increasing demands that accompany the growing geriatric population. Moreover, there is evidence to suggest that such legal intervention into familial relationships often leads to more harm than good. In particular, many adult children today face the conflicting demands of responsibility to their aging parents on the one hand and responsibility to their own children on the other. Alliances and loyalties can tug from each end and it would clearly be unfair of society to mandate sacrifice and support of an elderly parent if it were to come at the expense of a child's future welfare.

As with resource allocation, society has yet to achieve consensus about appropriate levels of familial responsibility in caring for the elderly. While historical, religious, and personal value traditions underscore the bonds that tie families together, such traditions are sorely tested in the face of increasingly complex and sophisticated needs and demands. Is it reasonable to expect a working mother, with her own familial obligations, to undertake, in her "spare" time, the responsibility for seeing to the welfare of her aging parents as well? Debate has begun on the moral arguments to support and oppose such responsibilities. It is only likely to grow more heated and divisive, however, as we strive as a society to develop humane, just, and morally acceptable solutions, which do not, in the process, bankrupt the future of generations to come.

FOR DISCUSSION

1. While ours is a society that considers life precious and sacred, there are many who argue that certain fates are worse than death and that certain "qualities of life" are not worth living. Would it be possible to construct a social policy to accommodate both of these views and, in particular, one that could pave the way for certain persons to have their lives ended when conditions became unbearable for them? In concrete terms, what would such a policy look like? What would be the benefits and risks?

2. When, if ever, can we justify paternalistic interventions into the lives of elderly persons? Who should determine what level of risk is appropriate for an elderly person to undertake? Should different levels of activity require different "demonstrations" of autonomy, as defined by Miller? What level of deliberation or decision making should be demonstrated in the context of refusals of life-prolonging interventions?

3. Are there arguments to support the vast expenditures of resources during the last few months of an elderly person's life? Are such expenditures "owed" to elderly persons as a type of "reward" for reaching advanced age? Should considerations about future productivity and "value" to self or society be considered in the allocation of resources, such that it makes more sense to devote health care dollars to preventative efforts in younger populations?

4. Certain theories concerned with familial relationships argue a theme of reciprocity: that is, children are in the debt of their parents and are obligated to provide for their parents because of the life and upbringing their parents provided for them. Comment on this perspective regarding the responsibility of adult children to provide fiscal, physical, or emotional support for their aging and ailing elderly parents.

REFERENCES

Beauchamp, T. L., and Childress, J. F. *Principles of Biomedical Ethics* (2nd edition). New York: Oxford University Press, 1983.

Brody, Baruch A., and Englehardt, H. Tristam. *Bioethics: Readings and Cases.* Englewood Cliffs, N.J.: Prentice-Hall, Inc., 1987.

Callahan, D. *Setting Limits: Medical Goals in an Aging Society.* New York: Simon and Schuster, 1987.

Daniels, N. *Am I My Parents' Keeper?: An Essay on Justice Between the Young and the Old.* New York: Oxford University Press, 1988.

Kapp, M. B., Pies, H. E., and Doudera, A. E. *Legal and Ethical Aspects of Health Care for the Elderly.* Ann Arbor, Mich.: Health Administration Press, 1985.

Lesnoff-Caravaglia, Gari. *Values, Ethics and Aging.* New York: Human Sciences Press, Inc., 1985.

Macklin, Ruth. *Mortal Choices: Ethical Dilemmas in Modern Medicine.* Boston: Houghton Mifflin Company, 1987.

McKee, Patrick L. *Philosophical Foundations of Gerontology.* New York: Human Sciences Press, Inc., 1982.

Office of Technology Assessment, Congress of the United States. *Life-Sustaining Technology and the Elderly.* Washington, D.C.: U.S. Government Printing Office, OTA-BA-306, 1987.

Spicker, S. F., Ingman, S. R., and Lawson, I. R. *Ethical Dimensions of Geriatric Care.* Dordrecht, Holland: D. Reidel Publishing Company, 1987.

11

Love, Sex, and Marriage in the Later Years

Doris B. Hammond

MYTHS AND FACTS

Myths concerning sexuality have persisted throughout the history of Western culture. Of these many myths, perhaps the most difficult to dispel concern the sexual ability, activity, and interest of older persons. Our older citizens are often caught in the turmoil that these myths cause. Consider the following five myths that are specific to older adults:[1]

Myths

1. Older people do not have sexual desires.
2. Older people couldn't make love even if they wanted to.
3. Older people are so physically fragile that sex might hurt them.
4. Older people are physically unattractive and, therefore, sexually undesirable.
5. The whole notion of sex for older people is shameful and decidedly perverse.

Would an older person in your family agree with these myths? Do you agree with these myths? Let's look at the facts.

Facts

1. Older people do have sexual desires. We are sexual beings from birth to death. Although there may be decreases in levels of arousal and a lessening in intensity, along with a slowing down of response, older people desire the closeness and touching that is so much a part of humanness. Yes, grandma and grandpa still desire each other as much as they always have.

2. Why do we think older people couldn't make love even if they wanted to? Do we think they can no longer bake a cake? Swim? Read a book? Fix a car? Why do we think they cannot make love? Have they forgotten how? Or, perhaps, it is the judgment of society that they can't anymore and probably don't want to anyway? First of all, we know that they can and do make love. Sexual activity drops off in the sixties for women and in the seventies for men, but for many—especially those who have partners—there is little decrease. One wonders how much the self-fulfilling prophecy of the older years as "sexless" has caused this decrease. When these folks were younger they probably felt that people became "neutered" with age, so in their own old age they perpetuated the myth.

3. Older people are too fragile and sex might hurt them. On the contrary, sex helps older people both physically and psychologically. Only the very frail and those in extreme poor health seem to be nonresponsive. Sex can actually be therapeutic. It can relieve the pain of arthritis as it increases the output of cortisone. (For continued relief, however, it has been suggested that one would have to have sex every four hours!) Likewise, it is a great pain reliever for backaches. The older person who is sexually active needs fewer tranquilizers and antidepressants. Having sex has even been thought to add to longevity while encouraging a stronger sense of self. The psychological benefits of maintaining a sense of self have been documented throughout our life span.

Some people have the mistaken notion that sex can cause death, especially in older people. No greater percentage of deaths occur during intercourse than during any other activity that expends the same amount of energy. Even when intercourse is with a "secret" partner, the added stress this brings about causes little rise in the incidence of death. Perhaps the best advice is to keep in practice with sex, just as you keep in practice with tennis or any other activity.

4. Society (and we're part of it!) has really done a job on us with respect to viewing older people as physically unattractive and, therefore, sexually undesirable. This myth contains within it another myth: that only physically attractive people want to have sex with each other. There are a lot of physically unattractive (by society's standards) younger people who would disagree. Maybe someone who is attractive to you is not attractive to me: I may not want to have sex with him, but you might! This is what keeps all of us from wanting to have sex with the same person. Thank goodness! But to lump all older people into the category of being unattractive just because they are old is an insult. I might add that this myth is particularly hard on the older woman for she is the one more often judged as physically unattractive, whereas the older man is often considered still attractive, or distinguished at the very least.

5. Many older people feel that sexual thoughts of any kind are shameful, if not perverse. A growing number of the elderly are beginning to believe otherwise. It is children who have the hardest time accepting the sexuality of their parents and grandparents. In fact, a child's view of his or her parents' sexuality often takes a tougher line than the parents' view of their children's and adolescents' sexuality.

As a counter to the myth that older people are sexless or uninterested in sex, we have to be careful not to accept an opposing myth, which claims that older people are as interested in sex now as when they were young. The traditional norms were an escape from sex, but contemporary norms are a reflection of our culture's frantic search for the fountain of youth. Also, we must be careful not to impose sex upon those for whom it does not have top priority. Continuity of life is what we must strive for.

Normative expectations must be developed that separate youthful sex and aging sex without implying that one is a degenerative form of the other. Aging sex is quantitatively different from youthful sex and is to be enjoyed in and of itself. Older people too often become the object of jokes and are frequently ridiculed as "dirty old men" or "senile old women." Popular opinion has them steadily declining into oblivion. Even though the sexuality of older people is not identical to that of the young, their need for intimacy and sexual expression endures.

SOCIETAL INFLUENCES

Our values concerning how we think about sex and how we conduct ourselves as sexual beings are acquired in much the same way we acquire values that guide us in other areas of social life. They are acquired through the "ultimate authority" of sacred scripture, from parental authority figures, from education, from folk wisdom found in legends and old wives' tales, through common conversation, from jokes and cliche phrases, and from the media. From these authorities we adopt major assumptions about what is good and bad sexually, what is appropriate and inappropriate, and what incites pleasure or induces repugnance. These clusters of assumptions operate as sexual value systems and are internalized by our personality structure. Most of our values become set in place at or about the age of ten; they then change slowly, usually with great effort or at the prompting of a significant emotional event. It is important, therefore, that we recognize the influences that surround our older population when they were very young, from around the turn of the century to the 1930s.

Sexual decline that may occur in an older person is more an artifact of social prohibitions and partner availability than it is a biological factor. Although there are some cultural restrictions on the older male, his sexuality is primarily limited by physical capacity. Conversely, the older female is limited more by cultural factors than physical ones since aging does not substantially affect the sexual capacity of females, compared to males. The double standard remains alive and well as a cultural factor that can impede sexual fulfillment. There are many more widows than widowers. Women average more than a decade of widowhood because they will live more than seven years longer than their male counterparts and will have married someone approximately three years older than themselves. Biology plays cruel tricks on females, leaving a large army of women without partners. One trick that society plays is making it seem the "rule" that men should be older than the women they marry and then, in old age, making it all right for the few remaining older men to marry young women while deeming it inappropriate for older women to marry or have any sort of relationship with younger men.

Various solutions have been proposed. An obvious one is for a woman to marry a younger man. An added benefit of this suggestion would be that the two would be sexually more in tune, since a man reaches his sexual peak at age eighteen and a woman at age thirty (not a biological difference, but rather because it takes her longer to uncover the sexual self that society for so many years has determined she should repress). How about polygamy for women as a possible solution? Would homosexual relationships among women who did not previously exhibit that identity be a solution that society could support? Can we as a society recognize the need for human contact, caring, and touching as one that transcends any age or gender confinement? Society needs to take a closer look at age-discrepant relationships and alternative lifestyles, not as indicating psychopathology but rather as an emotionally healthy way to choose mates based upon psychological compatibility rather than social standards of propriety and normalcy. How we address ourselves to these and other issues will have a great deal to do with how we grow as a society and how we express our own sexuality.

The social world in which today's elderly grew up would not have allowed them to examine what has been suggested in the previous paragraph. Even the most "liberated" knew little of the "facts of life," and most held to strong superstitions and to a puritan ethic. They were greatly affected by the Victorian era. It certainly wasn't a healthy climate for exploring sexual problems. In fact, it was totally inappropriate for examining problems of any sort through open communication. Everything was to be left within the family. Never "wash your linen in public" was the creed of the day. With the family failing to communicate about sexual problems, they remained hidden. Family members still have difficulty talking about sex with each other. Sex remains a mystery. No wonder those who lived during the previous eras are often shocked when presented with ways of solving the mystery of sex, since sexual discussions had never really been a part of the family pow-wows.

Our society is careful to admonish older people to "act your age." This becomes a very real problem for older people who are not sure what this means. Whether actually heard from a family member or assumed through the conditioning of an age-conscious society, perhaps the only safe way to behave is to sit in a rocking chair. At least elders know what they are permitted to do, even if society sometimes thinks they are so old they can't even get it (the rocking chair) going. Each one would "act our age." When young we shouldn't act too old, when older we shouldn't act too young. When hearing an older man make a sexually suggestive remark, we think of him as either senile or a dirty old man. That same remark, made by a younger man, however, would be considered "macho." When we see an older woman dressed attractively and in good health and physical condition, we say she "looks young for her age." That is her age and that's how she looks at that age, not as a younger caricature of herself.

How often do we change the tone of our voice when we talk to older people? It's as though they have become children. This is the "kindergarten voice," the voice so often affected by kindergarten teachers when they talk to their pupils. Have you ever found yourself talking in a higher pitch and using simpler terms, as though the older person couldn't understand? What an insult! The logical end to this type of thinking is that we view elders as childish beings, playing house with each other, rather than as mature individuals expressing a sexual maturity gained through years of loving.

We live in an age of "isms." First we learned about racism and then about sexism. To this has been added another: ageism. As examples of prejudiced viewpoints and as awful as each is in its particulars, I would like to suggest that ageism is perhaps the most difficult of all to understand. Why? If we are racist, we will never be of another race; if we are sexist, we will never (with rare exceptions) be another sex. However, if we are ageist, we will, in the end (barring premature death), be the beneficiaries of our own ridiculous prejudice. Think about that the next time you make judgments based upon age. Remember that the only alternative to aging is death.

Have you noticed that all old people are thought of in the same way: old? Nothing else, just old. This includes the notion that all old people don't enjoy sex. Some don't, but some young people don't either. A mistake is made when stratifying people into groups by age and then identifying each individual as having all the characteristics we assign to his or her particular group.

Magazine covers continue to present their audiences with nubile young girls who look out at us in various stages of dress and undress, taunting us with a look that is sexy but who couldn't actually know what real sex is all about. They just haven't lived long enough. It's about time we see the middle-aged and older men and women looking at us with the wisdom of experiences in their eyes, being portrayed as sexual beings. The more covers of this nature, the more television programs like "The Golden Girls," the more sensitized society will become to the worth of its older citizens.

For years movies have used older actors and actresses in character roles only. Men, however, have always fared better. The list of names is endless of men who, in their "mature years," were still considered great lovers. Don't most women still adore Paul Newman? But what of older women? Either the well-known names have disappeared from the screen as though they no longer existed, or these actresses were saddled with sexless, often demented, roles. There are too many "Baby Janes"!

Even though beauty has been important to women and is equated with sexuality, women have been more sexually repressed than men in their family structure. The extent of the repression varies, but it is obvious even in old age.

It is easy to see how the relationship between elders and society and the latter's negative cues have had a strong impact on the self-concept of our older people. Sexuality is an integral part of one's self-concept. Since society prescribes sexlessness—and most of our older citizens were raised to respect the dictates of society—they take this prescription too well, and often without question. They struggle hard to learn behaviors that will hide their sexuality. Could that be why a mother who was usually a well-dressed, stylish lady changes to a drab, unkempt old woman who isolates herself from others and protects herself from negative reactions?

Finally, the strength of cultural expectations is made even more obvious by a reported study of 106 cultures.[2] Many of these cultures have expectations for continued sexual activity of older men and women and, as might be expected, that activity flourishes. Interestingly, many of these reports showed an expectation for greater sexual activity on the part of older women than older men. As one might expect, this is exactly what happened. Doesn't this show very clearly the strong effect that cultural expectations have on sexual behavior?

DEVELOPMENTAL SEXUALITY

Physical and emotional health affect the sexual responses of males earlier and more directly than is the case with females. Illness, strain, and anxiety lower the levels of the male hormone testosterone. The present picture for male sexual health is rather dismal and can only be improved with earlier education in sexuality and drastic changes in the socialization patterns of men. Unfortunately, even older men, to whom we ascribe maturity, have not gained adequate knowledge of sexual health or the wisdom to use it.

A recurring theme in the relevant literature depicts sexual enjoyment as a capacity developed early and one that can be maintained throughout life. There are physiological changes, but psychological elements are probably of far more consequence in determining the character of older people's sex drives.

The Duke (University) Longitudinal Studies have provided much needed data on sexual functioning in the middle and later years. Some generalizations of these results follow:

1. The older one gets the less heterosexual activity takes place, although men are more active than women at any age.

2. Sexual activity (especially among males) seems to decline sharply in the mid-seventies with the onset of debilitating illness.

3. The older the person the lower the degree of sexual interest.

4. Decreasing sexual activity and interest patterns occur earlier for women than for men.

5. Both men and women report awareness of sexual decline.

6. Cessation of sexual activity was primarily the result of male dysfunction (e.g., inability to achieve or maintain an erection, losing interest in sex, being too ill to engage in the sex act).

7. Marital status made a great difference in the sexual activity level for women, but less for men.[3]

Developmentally, changes do occur in women that can affect their sexuality. Changes in the genitals occur during the years after menopause. These include a gradual shrinking and atrophying of the uterus and constriction of the vaginal lining. Vaginal secretions, which lubricate in anticipation of and during intercourse, may diminish, resulting in pain (dyspareunia) during intercourse. There may be vaginal burning and itching. All of this sounds awful, but most women feel no discomfort and those who do simply need to see a physician for suggested treatment.

With respect to emotional changes in women as they age, several reasons explain why older women feel more sexual:

1. the elimination of any concern about pregnancy;

2. the children are reared and thus no longer likely to intrude on intimate moments;

3. the lower response of an aging partner may afford women more time for sexual pleasuring; and

4. there is an increase in time and energy available to the couple, especially after retirement.[4]

Some women, however, use the "excuse" of menopause or advancing years to avoid the personal embarrassment of what they are afraid is inadequate sexual performance. They may also be experiencing the frustration of unresolved sexual tensions. However, in nearly all instances of actual cessation of sexual intercourse, the responsibility rests with the male.

Men have more opportunity to satisfy their sexuality as they age: if married, they may opt for extramarital partners; if single or unattached, they can "play the field." In any case, however, they often feel the need to meet certain standards of performance, standards better suited for men thirty years their junior.

We often hear the term "male menopause" bandied about, but there really is no male condition (emotional or physical) that corresponds to female menopause. The male testes continue to function, although there is a gradual decline in the rate of testosterone and of sperm production. Men can continue to father children, but since the sperm count is lower, fertilization is not as frequent. Erectal impotence affects one of every four males at age seventy, whereas it affects only 1 percent of males at age thirty-five.[5] The correlation between aging and impotence, however, is not inevitable. It is important to remember that psychologically induced impotence can be treated, and several devices have been perfected to allow an erection for a man with physiologically induced impotence.

At around age sixty, men have an average of slightly less than one copulation with orgasm per week, whereas those age fifteen to twenty average four per week. The frequency of morning erections drops steadily with age. More stimulation is necessary to produce an erection and more time is needed to produce a second erection. A young man may be able to have a second erection almost immediately, whereas an older male might take up to twenty-four hours.[6] The force of the ejaculate is less and, therefore, may cause a decrease in sensation. There is also some decline of erotic response to sexual stimulation (those calendar girls don't excite as quickly or as intensely anymore). The older male may have a tendency to be more absorbed in work than in sex, until he retires. But then, look out! Often he will experience a renewed sexual drive once his work pressures are behind him.

There is no biological imperative for a sudden end to sexual activity. Overall reduction in vigor and strength may decrease sexual capacity but it does not result in an end to sexual activity for either men or women. Those who were most sexually active in their younger years will continue to be the most sexually active as they grow older.

Popular misconceptions about the needs and desires of older people continue to flourish, in spite of evidence to the contrary. It is the older people themselves who are becoming more vocal about the denial of their sexuality. It is doubtful they can ever escape the values of their own upbringing, but some are beginning to look at the possibilities that have been part of the sexual experience of other age groups, such as cohabitation, group living arrangements, and homosexual relationships.

Perhaps the sexual abilities and interest of older adults can best be summarized by two wonderful quotations from Alex Comfort, who can be counted among the old generation himself. He wrote the following in his book *The Joy of Sex:*

> The only thing age has to do with sex performance is that the longer you love, the more you learn. Young people (and some older ones) are finally convinced that no one over fifty makes love, and it would be pretty obscene if they did. Ours isn't the first generation to know otherwise, but probably the first one which hasn't been brainwashed into being ashamed to admit it!

> The best producer of an active and pleasurable sex life in the later years is an active and pleasurable sex life in the early years; the things that stop a person from having sex with increasing age are exactly the things that stop one from bicycle riding: bad health, thinking it looks silly, not having a bicycle. The difference is they happen later for sex than for bicycles.[7]

A small percentage of our elders have never married. A very small percentage of them will marry after age fifty. For the most part, those who have remained single (especially women), report few negative effects, though the adjustment to marriage may, in effect, be difficult for those who have remained single for many years.

If there were equal numbers of men and women in later years, most experts agree that women would be the more active sex. A woman's sex drive continues to grow until age thirty and then levels off throughout the remainder of her life. A man's sex drive peaks early, and progressively lessens; for some, it disappears altogether in advanced age.

FAMILY VIEWS OF OLDER MEMBERS' SEXUALITY

Family members accepting their elders as sexual beings is something most people have really never thought about. As parents we worry about teenage sexuality, but as children we rarely, if ever, think about the sexuality of our parents. An interesting study, conducted at Illinois State University, examined the feelings of 646 students regarding their parents' sexuality. The results showed that 90 percent of the students felt their parents were happily married and still in love; furthermore, they believed that their parents maintained this happy state without the help of sex, or at least not much of it. These results seemed both amusing and sad.

The image produced may be of two aging people who have loved each other for years, holding hands and smiling, perhaps gently kissing each other on the cheek. But could we imagine these same two elders lying in bed nude, having intercourse? Probably not! Not my mother and father! Certainly not my grandmother and grandfather! Very slowly, though, some deterioration of this psychological blockage is occurring. Bumper stickers now proclaim, "I'm not a dirty old man, I'm a sexy senior citizen."

Communication in families can affect childhood perceptions of adult sexuality. In families where there is open communication, children tend to feel that their parents have more sexual activity. Even for these children, though, it seems easier to imagine other older adults having sex rather than those in their own families. These offspring still report lower rates of presumed parental sexual intercourse or sexual intimacy of older adults than the actual rates of occurrence indicated by Kinsey's survey results or even more recent surveys.

Parental sexuality has probably been one of the most successfully kept secrets of all time. Children may find out the "secrets" of other family affairs, such as the income level or that Uncle Jim is gay, but it takes longer for them to arrive at the remarkable discovery that their parents must have had sex, at least enough times to produce one offspring and maybe a sibling or two. But since that brings a shudder of disbelief, they would prefer not to think there were many more times than absolutely necessary. It usually is a little easier to think of Dad as having sex, since that is expected of men, than it is to think of Mom. That's almost unpatriotic and a blemish on the character of the very person who is synonymous with apple pie and all that is good in the world. Here, again, is the idea that sex is dirty and Mom must remain untainted by anything "evil."

Sex education classes are offered for the young but not for the middle-aged or the old. This leads one to believe that the only purpose of education is to provide information about birth control. It keeps sex tied to procreation and not the sexual expression of loving people who happen to be beyond the age of reproduction. As parents we are, or should be, concerned about all aspects of sex education for our children. Wouldn't it be a significant step forward if we became concerned about our parents' sex education and even our own? Can we imagine a time in the future when our children would sign us up for sex education classes? The fact that we have had children evidences little correlation with what we know about sex, given the large amount of misinformation we pass on to our children.

There are many older people who could really educate their families about sex if relatives would only ask. One elder said that her children know about her sexual liaisons and she finds their reactions to her lifestyle very interesting. Their major concern seems to be that she might get hurt or be too generous with her material possessions.

What if this elder wanted to remarry? What are the reactions of families to the remarriage of a parent or grandparent? Single or widowed parents who live with younger relatives are often made to feel guilty, if not indecent, for even wanting to date. Yet men and women are getting married—or remarried—in increasing numbers. Recent studies tell us that in a single year there are more than 16,000 brides and 33,000 grooms who are sixty-five years of age or older. Most couples who marry in their later years report that they had to overcome the objections and concerns of their children, their friends, or both.

Our culture often frowns upon late marriages. Perhaps those children who seek to prevent the marriage of an elderly widow or widower are afraid of losing an inheritance, or they may think it is unseemly. Elders who are themselves concerned about fairness with respect to financial matters, might deal with this by carefully preparing their wills so that assets prior to their marriage remain their own and anything that accrues after their marriage becomes joint property. This seems fair in light of the contributions that were made when a previous spouse was living.

As for the unseemly part of remarriage or of sexual intimacy, adult children can assume the major portion of blame when they view their elders' normal urges for intimacy, romance, and commitment as evidence of a second childhood and therefore cause for social disgrace. Many children are much more comfortable suggesting that their parents or grandparents take up a hobby or become more involved in their families, that the elders provide household and baby-sitting services, rather than encourage them to enter the mainstream of life through an intimate relationship. Some of this intolerance for parental sexuality may stem from hidden resentment caused by repressed childhood feelings regarding sexual needs that went unfulfilled: "If you didn't let me why should I let you?" Their parents may seem to be acting in a sexually liberated way in which they as children had never been permitted to indulge.

As families become more mobile, often with members living considerable distances from each other, this preoccupation with the sexuality of a family member is beginning to dissipate. The mobile elderly are able to free themselves from the "good will" of their offspring when it comes to sexual activity, much like what happens when a child leaves home.

The expression of love is a human need shared by all family members; it should not be based upon the number of years one has lived. Family members need to realize that each individual is a sexual being from birth until death. Obviously that does not mean having intercourse at birth, or in early childhood. "Sexual being," therefore, means something far more encompassing than intercourse. In our Western society we might describe this in terms of love. That is a major part of our sexuality—expressing love and being able to love someone else. Reaching out to someone, touching, and caring, all of these add to our sense of self. No matter how old, each family member deserves the dignity that being fully human requires of all who live in civilized society.

HEATH AND SEXUALITY

The search for a fountain of youth and the human desire to live to a ripe old age have provided a mixed bag of positive and negative results. As we dramatically increase life expectancy through better medical care and nutrition, we increase the possibility of illness during those additional years. The longer we live, the more chance there is for disability.

Unfortunately, if society deems the old to be asexual, think how this is compounded by being disabled. The facts of human physiology and statistical probability over time increase the chances for this combination to occur. The older we are the less resistance we have to illness, the longer it takes to recuperate, and the greater the incidence of chronic disease.

Since good health is significantly related to feelings of pleasure and satisfaction, our state of mind can have an enormous impact on the state of our health.

Many people believe that illness marks the beginning of the end of sexual activity. To a degree this is true: the trauma of disease causes the body to summon up energy to fight off illness and thus little energy is left for sexual outlets. A chronic illness can produce the same effect but for a much longer period of time.

Recovery from acute illness may be sufficiently rapid, therefore not altering the patient's sense of sexual self and his or her level of sexual activity can be resumed with little or no interruption. Chronic illness may produce greater levels of anxiety as the patient learns to "live with" and adjust to the permanence of a disability. Illness, accident, or surgery may cause an alteration in a patient's concept of his or her body image. This may require a supportive family, a supportive sexual partner, and a sympathetic physician who is willing to deal with sexual matters. Counseling may also be needed; in fact, it should probably be considered an indispensable part of the recovery process.

Even though impaired health may affect sexual functioning, it must be remembered that old age by itself causes a slowed response. Some studies have indicated that declines in sexual activity are related more to aging than to health. The two factors together produce the greatest effect. Aging itself is a disease state only if we allow it to be. However, there is a greater chance of actual health problems in old age.

Sexuality, including intercourse, has been found to have a positive effect on the health, both physical and mental, of older persons. Some studies indicate that it even increases life expectancy. Exercise in general has been known to do that, and sex is a form of exercise. Some disagree that there is an increase in life expectancy, but all agree that the quality of life is improved when we express our sexuality in some way. When we are in ill health, probably more than at any other time, we need the warmth, caring, and touching that affirms us as human beings.

Nursing home placement often signifies the end to sexual expression. Many concerned family members conscientiously use check lists to help them determine the quality of a nursing home they are considering. I have seen some very fine check lists prepared for that purpose, but rarely have I seen one that indicates anything about sexual privacy. When considering sexual needs, nursing home residents are truly a forgotten and neglected population. Unlike the general population in which most sexual activity takes place behind closed doors, those who reside in nursing homes are living in glass houses. Probably more often than we realize, sexual activity is taking place, but think of the clandestine maneuvering this involves and the subsequent feelings of guilt.

Nursing homes can deprive residents of their sexual rights, and many lead celibate lives. Residents are separated by gender and only permitted to mingle in the dining hall or lounge. Future generations, who were used to coed dormitories will have something to say about this when some of them enter nursing homes. The problem probably will take care of itself by that time, but why should residents have to wait for such liberation? At least the separation of married couples is becoming less frequent, unless they request to be separated (as some have done). But even when married couples occupy the same room, are they provided with a double bed as they have been used to? Of course not! The usual single beds suffice for everyone. Not only is nighttime the best, and perhaps only, time for couples to snuggle together, but if they both have to get into a single bed in order to do it, it's a real safety hazard!

Sexual history is often overlooked in medical and nursing home records. One home's admission form did not include a sexual history until a troubled eighty-two-year-old man wondered why nothing had been asked about his sex life. He said this was important to him and that he had been having some problems lately. After taking a sexual history, the physician learned valuable information.

Are too many nursing home practices geared to institutional efficiency and the desires of the families rather than the patients themselves? Some activists have suggested that it should be possible to sue a nursing home for not allowing sexual activity: the suit would be based upon a violation of civil rights. Even if unsuccessful, such suits would serve to stimulate an awareness of the issues pertaining to patient rights. Until there are more advocates to make the concerns of nursing home residents highly visible, this probably will not happen. Nursing home residents tend, instead, to be among the most powerless, voiceless, and invisible groups in our country.

Many nursing home patients suffer from chronic anxiety, a condition that can be relieved by sexual orgasm. Enlightened staff and administrators of nursing homes, realizing the therapeutic value of sex, may knowingly turn their backs on clandestine sexual liaisons or solitary sexual behavior. A few actually encourage the activity. One said he wished there was more of it. When questioned as to why there wasn't, he said it was mainly a problem for the staff.

Some nursing homes have set aside designated "petting rooms" where residents can go for privacy. This seems a little contrived, however, and those who choose to go there would probably feel that all eyes are upon them and might expect to hear both staff and fellow residents say, "We know where you're going!"

Beyond designating rooms for use by residents who desire to be intimate, some administrators have arranged for in-service education for the staff, whose feelings are a reflection of every social attitude. On one end are those who feel that whatever someone wants to do is perfectly all right with them, provided it is not hurting someone else. On the other end are the "protectors of us all" who feel it is their moral duty to control the behavior of others, based upon what they believe is right.

Patient education programs should be implemented to discuss topics ranging from medical problems to atrophy resulting from sexual disuse. This could develop from an unstructured group setting and eventually expand to include discussions about sexuality after the group becomes comfortable with the leader. This would be better than starting right off talking about sex. Residents need to gain a better understanding and respect for the sexual needs of others. Often, through jealousy, they condemn the actions of others or, like some staff, they are on the end of the continuum that says you must live by my moral standards. One staff member did mention that she considers the jealousy of other residents to be a primary inhibitor of sexual activity.

It is very probable that some residents of nursing homes have a greater need than others for sexual intimacy. For those already suffering from a disability, emotional closeness can be of considerable benefit to their self-concept and self-esteem. Encouragement can be given in this area by helping residents to dress more attractively, thereby helping them to feel better about themselves. When residents feel better about themselves, they also feel better about each other. Even the reaction of staff to eye-appealing residents results in more time being spent with them. The individual sense of masculinity and femininity is thus maintained and possibly enhanced.

ENHANCING SEXUALITY

Older couples can be helped to understand their sexuality if they recognize that normal age-related changes do exist, that they are not the same for the male and the female, and that each person reacts to changes in his or her special way. These changes are biological processes, none of which are produced by the quality of the couple's love or by their individual attractiveness. The presence of problems need not have any permanent affect on sexual functioning, provided they are discussed in an atmosphere of love, acceptance, and openness. Even the intimacy of intercourse can be set aside if individuals who are physically and spiritually close are able to find other ways to show tenderness, love, and respect for each other.

There are many things elders can do to understand and remedy sexual, personal, and social problems. Reading books and other related materials could be a starting point. Viewing films, attending lectures, taking part in workshops, all can be of benefit. Enrolling in a human sexuality class is a good idea. A course listing at local colleges and universities should help interested persons find the right class, most of which can be audited. Obtaining a thorough medical examination, and being willing to mention any sexual problems or concerns to the physician, is absolutely necessary. Physical problems can combine with social and emotional problems and eventually manifest themselves in a wide array of symptoms indicating sexual dysfunction. When problems persist, a counselor can be of tremendous help. Beyond expertise in matters physical, a physician cannot be expected to offer advice; a counselor should step in here when psychological problems present themselves.

Counseling can be on an individual or group basis. Group counseling may be more conducive to exploration and sharing. In a group session members can support each other while exploring sensitive feelings. Older individuals, however, have not experienced groups as much as the youth of today. Therefore, they may feel more comfortable with the privacy of individual counseling. For some older persons who grew up at a time when schoolroom desks were bolted to the floor in straight lines, group work, especially in such delicate and personal matters, is not for them.

Older males who seek counseling may be experiencing a type of monotony brought on by being with the same partner or doing things the same way. If not yet retired, they may be preoccupied with their careers. Some may be experiencing mental or physical fatigue, physical infirmity, or the disability of their partners. Perhaps overindulging in food or drink is the culprit. Then, of course, there is always the possibility of anxiety over performance—the old "fear of failure" syndrome. Some older persons may have become too inattentive to their own personal appearance, resulting in sloppiness, careless personal hygiene, or obesity. Here exercise and controlled diet are of paramount importance.

Since women have been conditioned to equate desirability with youth and beauty, their responsiveness can be affected to the extent that they perceive themselves to be old and ugly. A counselor can't change the "old," but she (I would suggest a woman counselor here) can help an older woman to be more attractive through exercise and good grooming followed by working on her ability to see herself as attractive. Much of the decline in sexual interest among aging women is not physiological but defensive. Many find it more adaptive to inhibit sexual strivings when little opportunity exists for sexual fulfillment.

It is important for older men and women to maintain or develop a pattern of sexual activity congruent with their own needs and with the aging process. There must be open and honest communication that is sensitive to the wishes of others. This includes the ability of each partner to verbalize his or her expectations. Each needs to explore avenues of sexual pleasure without intercourse and to consider alternate positions that are more effective for stimulating and maintaining an erection. The couple might try mutual masturbation as a variation on, or addition to, their "usual" lovemaking repertoire.

Counselors must be careful not to impose current cultural expectations upon older clients, a group who cannot be expected in any immediate way to overcome the sexual misapprehensions and taboos with which they have lived for so long. It is important not to put someone in conflict with his or her own values by enforcing the counselor's personal morality and convictions. Since sexual performance in older persons is predicted by their performance throughout life, it must be kept in mind that for those older people who were not sexually active when young, a satisfactory involvement at another age may be far less active than for someone else, and yet every bit as satisfying.

Sexual therapy, since its inception, has been of a conjoint nature, the assumption being that there are two persons in need of counseling. In the case of older women, however, this type of therapy has no value for those who are alone. For this group, counseling to deal with aloneness is very much in order. Great sensitivity is required if such women are to be informed of the various options available and also helped to affirm themselves as women.

Those with health problems need information to be shared regarding health or disability. There are many practical ways to assist a couple. For the stroke victim, a football or trapeze will assist mobility. An arthritic may enjoy early morning sex preceded by a hot bath as part of foreplay to loosen joints. Those who complain that aspirin reduces sexual sensation should have sex before taking the medication. Use of a lubricant is most helpful for the woman who has reduced vaginal secretions. Don't bother taking an aphrodisiac: many older people (and younger ones as well) have tried this route, but the Food and Drug Administration has assured us that the myriad claims of obtaining super sexual status are sheer myth. So, forget about wine, Spanish fly, cayenne pepper, snakeroot, bloodroot, Vitamin E, and marijuana. The only true aphrodisiacs are good diet, good exercise, and a vivid imagination.

Sex should not be thought of as a prescription for what ails us, but rather as part of our total sexuality. Those who have developed a lifestyle that does not include the first three letters in sexuality should not be made to feel guilty, as though they have not taken an essential vitamin. Likewise, those who have maintained sex as part of their total sexuality should feel society's acceptance of this as a very normal part of their lives. What elders need in order to feel sexual and sensual is an acceptance and love of their own bodies, a zest for life in general, and an appreciation of the sexuality and sensuality of others. Is that any different from what is needed at any age? Of course not!

NOTES

1. Butler, R. N., and Lewis, M. I., *Aging and Mental Health* (St. Louis, Mo.: 1977), p. 112.
2. Winn, R., and Newton, N., "Sexuality in Aging: A Study of 106 Cultures," *Archives of Sexual Behavior* 11 (1982): 283–98.
3. Pfeiffer, E., Verwoerdt, A., and Dairs, G. C., "Sexual Behavior in Middle Life," *American Journal of Psychiatry* 128 (1972): 82–87.
4. Barbach, L., *For Yourself: The Fulfillment of Female Sexuality* (New York: Doubleday and Company, 1975), p. 2.
5. Katchadourian, H. A., and Lund, D. T., *Fundamentals of Human Sexuality.* 2d ed. (New York: Holt Rinehart and Winston, 1975), p. 371.
6. Sadock, B. J., Kaplan, H. I., and Friedman, A. M., *The Sexual Experience* (Baltimore: The Williams and Wilkins Company, 1976).
7. Comfort, A., *The Joy of Sex* (New York: Crown Publishers, 1972), p. 224.

FOR DISCUSSION

1. What are some of the myths about sexuality and aging? Can you name some others you have heard?
2. How does society affect the sexuality of men and women in different ways?
3. What physical changes affect the sexuality of men? Of women?
4. What are barriers to the expression of sexuality in institutions?

BIBLIOGRAPHY

Anderson, B. G. *The Aging Game: Success, Sanity, and Sex After Sixty.* New York: McGraw-Hill, 1985.
Bowtin, C. *Is There Sex After Marriage?* Boston: Little Brown & Co., 1985.
Brecher, E. M., and Eds. of Consumer Report Books. *Love, Sex and Aging.* Boston: Little Brown and Co., 1984.
Butler, R. N., and Lewis, M. I. *Sex After Sixty: A Guide for Men and*

Women for Their Later Years. New York: Harper and Row, 1976.

Comfort, A. *The Joy of Sex*. New York: Crown, 1976

Gochros, H. L., Grochros, J. S., and Fischer, J. (eds.). *Helping the Sexually Oppressed*. Englewood Cliffs, N.J.: Prentice-Hall, 1986.

Hammond, D. *My Parents Never Had Sex*. Buffalo, N.Y.: Prometheus Books, 1987.

Partnow, E. *Breaking the Age Barrier*. New York: Pinnacle Books, 1981.

Porcino, J. *Growing Older, Getting Better: A Handbook for Women in the Second Half of Their Life*. Reading, Mass.: Addison-Wesley Publishing Co., 1983.

Solnick, R. L. (ed.). *Sexuality and Aging*. Los Angeles: The University of Southern California Press, 1978.

Starr, B. D., and Weiner, M. B. *Sex and Sexuality in the Mature Years*. New York: Stein and Day, 1981.

Weg, R. B. (ed.). *Sexuality in the Later Years*. Orlando, Fla.: Academic Press, 1983.

12

Loss, Death, and Living

Deborah Wilkinson-Tjoa

One of the most important tasks of the elderly is to deal with a multitude of losses including the most significant, that of one's own life. With support, older people cope very well and can add great wisdom and understanding to all our lives if given the opportunity. Their last days can be a real gift in terms of the wealth of experiences and understandings they can share. What privilege it is to be at the transition, helping to witness life completing its purpose. How important are the lessons the dying can teach about living.

LOSSES

Throughout life we deal with many types of losses. Elizabeth Kübler-Ross, a psychiatrist at the forefront in the study of death, dying, and loss, calls these losses mini deaths. There are two categories of losses: situational and maturational. These losses in turn create other losses, resulting in a multitude of losses. Maturational losses are generally more predictable. They are closely related to the developmental stages identified by Erickson, which are

1. trust versus mistrust

2. autonomy versus shame and doubt

3. initiative versus guilt

4. industry versus inferiority

5. ego identity versus role confusion

6. intimacy versus isolation

7. generativity versus despair

Maturational Losses

These include

birth

infancy

childhood

adolescence

leaving home

marriage

the empty nest.

Birth is the loss of a protective environment for the baby and a loss of independence for the mother. During pregnancy, the mother is the focus of attention. When the baby is born, it becomes the focus of attention and the mother becomes tied to meeting the needs of the *infant,* resulting in a loss of her independence. The loss of *childhood* is often not addressed. How many people still remember who told them about Santa Claus not really being "there"? The mental health impact of the loss of childhood is significant since suicides have been reported in children as young as three.

The trials and tribulations of *adolescence* have long been identified. It is a time of reversals from dependence to independence. Finding "oneself" is a difficult task, often taking a lifetime. Trying to figure it all out in a brief period of time can cause great stress. The difficulties of adolescence have been documented by the severe problem of the second largest group to commit or attempt suicide.

Leaving home to go to school, or out on one's own is another loss, as is *marriage,* which leaves a person even more on his own.

Although *the empty nest* can signal a tremendous "freeing" experience, it can be another difficult transition. If most of one's time and energy went into taking care of the children, and little time was spent on activities geared towards self-satisfaction or constructive use of time, the impact of the loss would be more devastating.

Situational Losses

Losses that happen in a less predictable fashion are called situational. Examples include

  loss of school friends when changing grades

  loss of ideals (Santa Claus)

  loss of parents

  loss of work

  loss of a mate

  loss of a home (from natural to financial causes)

  burnout (actual or perceived loss of skills)

  loss of personal freedom

  loss of finances

  loss of bodily functions and/or body parts

  loss of one or more senses

  loss of independence

  loss of feeling useful and productive

  loss of friends

  loss of familiar surroundings

  loss of transportation

  loss of health

  loss of one's life

As can be seen, a situational loss triggers other losses. Maturational losses can trigger situational losses. Situational losses can trigger maturational losses.

WHY IDENTIFY LOSSES?

How we deal with losses very much affects how we age and how we will face death. Erickson proposes that as each stage of development is met, its result will affect the next stage. The task of the older person is to reach the state of integrity instead of despair. However, if the first stage, "autonomy versus shame," resulted in shame, it will be difficult for the older persons to reach integrity unless work is done with past events.

Each of us is unique. This individuality becomes more apparent as we age. We respond in special ways to our losses and therefore develop a pattern that is "our" pattern, our "grieving." Understanding the losses and changes that cause the most difficulty is important.

In today's society the highest rate of divorce occurs in the postretirement period. Divorce has been identified by the aged as one of the most difficult losses to resolve. This could be due, in part, to the lack of expectation. Most people in this age group have been married for twenty to thirty years at least. The elderly had anticipated that their later years would be a period of enjoyment and of spending time together. After the divorce, friends change, moving is generally indicated, and relationships with children, as well as those with other family members, become strained or changed. This, too, is a loss. Finances become involved and generally, especially for the female, this results in a loss of resources. Loss of this resource is difficult, if not impossible, to overcome. Employment for older women is unlikely.

Loss of ideals is also difficult. While planning one's life, the retirement years are seen as a time to travel and engage in leisure time activities. If a spouse becomes ill, this will culminate in disappointment and resentment. The loss is especially hard if the couple has put off enjoying their life until retirement.

EFFECTIVE GRIEVING

Although grieving can be very painful, it is a natural healing process. It helps us to come to a point where adjustment to the loss is possible. Satisfactory completion of loss does not, however, mean that significant losses will be gone and forgotten. Memories will return again and again: on holidays, birthdays, and other special occasions. Places associated with the event, certain smells, music, or sounds can remind us of the loss, and grief will ensue. The intensity will diminish, but it will be present.

Factors that influence grief include timing, significance of the loss, the person's history and philosophy of life.

Timing has been found to be an important factor affecting predictability and preparedness. Repeated studies have shown that if a person recognizes or expects the loss, the subsequent period of mourning is less intense and generally briefer in duration. Sudden and unexpected losses tend to be much more difficult and lengthy. Some insight into dealing with expected grief was identified in the 1940s by L. Lindeman, a psychiatrist. He found that women who expected their husbands to die in World War II went through an intense period of grieving. When the husbands returned, the relationship did not work out. He called this "anticipatory grieving." The women had already grieved the loss of the husbands and the relationships had effectively died.

Anticipatory grieving is done in many aspects of aging. Perhaps by grieving the change of residence before it occurs or anticipating the loss of a car, the person could overcome the change. This is only if the person has had time to anticipate these losses before they occur. Time is the important element in anticipatory grief. When an elderly person has a prolonged life-threatening illness, anticipatory grief will facilitate the grief response. However, where there is a prolonged illness and an older person taking care of the spouse, anticipatory grief doesn't necessarily occur. This could be owing to the length of time involved and to denying oneself both the time and the permission to grieve.

The significance of the loss strongly affects the intensity and duration of the grief period. It can also trigger many other losses that compound the grieving. For example, the death of a wife may trigger other losses, including those of a confidante, a lover, a person who buys and prepares meals, a person who straightens up the house, and a true friend. Making the move to a facility can trigger losses of territory and identification with memories, pieces of furniture, or pictures. Loss of independence resulting in nursing home placement and loss of health can also trigger grief.

A person's history helps to shape how that person will grieve. Many studies have shown that young children who lose a parent will have a more depressive outlook. Frequently, they will be treated for depression in later years. The pattern will become a blueprint. By surviving many losses and coping with them, a stability and strength will develop. Nietzsche once wrote "That which does not kill me makes me stronger." It is this strength from coping that increases the vitality of some people. Yet many persons are denied this opportunity to learn coping skills and are over-protected. They are seen as too frail to handle information of their ensuing loss or the death of someone close.

What a person *believes* contributes to how he relates to losses. For example, spiritual values are the "should's" and "should not's"; if a person believes that all things happen for the best, then the losses will be grieved but the tragedy may not be fully experienced according to others' values. If the person's philosophy is "life is unfair and bad things happen to me," then most losses will be perceived as bad and a terrible occurrence. Grief will be more profound.

THE PROCESS OF GRIEF

Many aspects of grieving have been identified (e.g., see Kübler-Ross, Kalish, Kastenbaum, Dixon). They are helpful in identifying some of the ways that peoples' patterns of grieving unfold. It must be kept in mind, however, that there are no stages. People may experience one emotion for a long time, or emotions may be constantly changing.

This process includes but is not necessarily limited to shock, denial, anger, rage, depression, guilt, fear, and resolution. Shock relates to the surprise of the loss. Regardless of one's preparedness, when the loss does actually come, there is surprise. Denial of the loss or its potential occurrence is quite common. Some people cope by continuing to deny the loss. They may use fantasy to cope with the loss rather than acknowledge or face it.

Anger is also a common way to express grief. This can be a difficult task if the persons have not been given, or do not grant themselves, permission to express this emotion. The anger is free floating, so many do not understand where to direct it. It can be directed toward the self or toward other people or things. Rage has been identified as a major emotion felt in the bereavement process. Dylan Thomas writes: "Do not go gently into that good night, old age should burn and rave at close of day; rage, rage against the dying of the light." Catherine Fanslow and Elizabeth Kübler-Ross suggest positive ways of letting out rage and anger. These include using a hose wrapped with toweling to hit a bed or pillow, twisting egg cartons, writing about the anger, or screaming. It is important to recognize the anger and to allow its expression.

Depression is perhaps the most prevalent emotion when facing loss. It is the most common psychiatric diagnosis, perhaps due to the grief reactions of people stuck in this stage. Crying is associated with both emotional and mental processes. It is interesting to note that tears of grief are different from tears of joy. Tears of grief have a higher level of toxicity and salt. The ramification is that grief is a physiological process. Sighing is another physical manifestation of grief. There is a high correlation of death from pneumonia after frail-aged people were relocated, mostly against their will. Tao, an ancient Chinese philosopher, stated that grief is held in the lungs. Yoga breathing techniques have been used successfully in ameliorating this problem and in helping to alleviate depression. Physical activity that enhances the respiratory process has been found successful in facilitating relief of depression in the overall grief process.

Feelings of fear and guilt are also natural when confronting a loss. Many fears develop with anxiety that swells and abates. Some people may then choose to live their lives in fear. Similar to guilt, these fears may or may not have a foundation. Guilt is often a painful thing to experience and difficult to help dissipate. In grief work, the "if only I had's" are all too familiar.

Resolution is not a static stage. A person may feel that a particular loss is resolved, only to find a holiday or special date approaching, hear a favorite song on the radio, or catch a whiff of that familiar cologne; and suddenly one is catapulted right back into the grief process.

It is important to respect and understand the process of bereavement for all of us eventually experience it: not just the older person, but the families and the counselors who take care of them. It is a dynamic process as individualized as a thumb print or DNA structure. Its progression can be facilitated by recognition of its facets and by carefully monitoring the ingestion of alcohol and drugs. Alcohol is a depressant and will therefore cause depression. Caffeine causes hostility and irritability and will subsequently make anger and rage more pronounced. Drugs, especially tranquilizers, antidepressants, and sedatives (which alter the REM sleep pattern), also alter the natural progression of healing. Dreamwork has been identified by the American Psychiatric Society as "important" in grieving. Dreaming about and perceptions of being with the person who has died are therapeutic. Alcohol, caffeine, and drugs can affect this dreamwork state and, in so doing, stifle the process.

Physical complaints and identification with the physical problems of the deceased are very common components in bereavement. Older persons come to physicians with symptoms similar to those experienced by the person who has died. The astute physician may well identify the grieving process, thereby encouraging the person to deal with the pain of grief. Sometimes this is a difficult task, since there often is the expectation that the pain can be circumvented.

The older person may discuss seeing the deceased person. This too is common. Psychiatric tests fail to validate this as an hallucination or delusion, for often it is accompanied by rational thoughts and acts. Mostly these "encounters" offer the bereaved some solace and should not be viewed as pathological or unnatural.

It cannot be stressed enough that there are no rigid stages or specific time frames for each step. This is important to acknowledge, since health professionals have punished patients for not reaching a state which the former believes the latter should have reached. "Punishment" results in withholding understanding, compassion, and respect. The duration, depth, and extent of the grieving process depend in large measure on the nature of the loss and its timeliness. Integration and resolution will depend upon the persons, their history, and their philosophy.

WHAT ARE THE PROBLEMS IN DEALING WITH THE AGED IN AREAS OF LOSS AND DEATH?

Cohen (1976) identifies three areas that counselors need to identify in assessing their values toward the aged:

1. The aged stimulate the counselor's fear of aging and death. In these instances, identifying the recognition of losses and permission to grieve these losses—especially death—are anxiety producing for the counselor. This will not be a healthy, caring, therapeutic milieu for the aged.

2. The elderly arouse the counselor's unresolved conflicts regarding parent figures. Although this identifies the dynamics of counter transference, it also demonstrates that the counselor cannot accept the individuality of the aged person and his/her specific needs.

3. The counselor believes he/she has nothing to offer because the older person will not be able to get better and will die anyway. With this judgmental behavior, improvement or ability to help the aged person is highly unlikely.

These values are important in the counselor's ability to work constructively with the aged. It is imperative that the counselor be open to (1) discussing loss and death, (2) identifying each older person and his/her family members as individuals, (3) respecting each person's ability to change, and (4) acknowledging the right to be treated with respect regardless of meeting or not meeting his/her value structure.

If fear of personal loss and subsequent death exists, how can a counselor effectively deal with the loss and death of another? This is a major dilemma, since few schools where counselors are trained have courses in loss or death and dying. Those institutions that have such courses do not require them for the health care professionals and counselors in the geriatric field.

SUICIDE

Alcohol consumption and suicide may be precipitated by a significant loss. There is a high correlation between the use of alcohol and incidents of suicide. White males over the age of seventy-five commit the most suicides. In particular, elderly widowers are the highest population at risk (Osgood 1985).

TABLE 1
UNITED STATES SUICIDE BY AGE AND SEX, 1978

Five-Year Suicide Rates

Age Group	Male	Female
5-9	0.0	0.0
10-14	1.2	0.4
15-19	12.8	3.1
20-24	27.4	6.4
25-29	27.5	7.9
30-34	23.4	8.3
35-39	22.3	9.3
40-44	21.4	11.0
45-49	22.5	11.1
50-54	24.3	11.3
55-59	25.4	10.8
60-64	30.1	8.4
65-69	30.2	8.3
70-74	37.2	7.4
75-79	45.9	8.4
80-84	50.6	6.0
85+	48.3	5.1

SOURCE: Elderly Suicide Data Bases: Levels, Availability, Omission (p. 19) by J. L. McIntosh. Paper presented at the Annual Meeting of the Gerontological Society of America, San Francisco, California, November, 1983. Reprinted with permission.

Assessing the potential for suicides, particularly in those males recently bereaved, is important. Cohen (1976) has found that the older male does tell someone of his intentions. This is generally the physician. Physicians, however, lack knowledge and experience in psychiatric assessments. They have been demonstrated to have little regard for mental health services. Unfortunately, then, the pleas or the cues go unrecognized.

When working with those believed to be potentially suicidal, it is important to ask them if they are thinking of harming themselves. If the answer is affirmative, it is important to ascertain if they have a plan. Despite the myth that asking about a plan forces the person to create a plan, the reality is that most suicidal persons will discuss the plan. Suicide among the aged has the same dynamics as among any other age group. The person sees with tunnel vision, obscuring the possibility of alternatives. Suicide

TABLE 2
UNITED STATES SUICIDE BY AGE AND RACE

Five-Year Suicide Rates

Age Group	White	Nonwhite
5–9	0.0	0.0
10–14	0.9	0.5
15–19	8.7	4.5
20–24	17.5	13.8
25–29	17.9	15.4
30–34	16.2	12.2
35–39	16.2	11.9
40–44	17.2	8.4
45–49	17.8	8.7
50–54	18.7	8.4
55–59	19.1	6.4
60–64	19.7	7.6
65–69	19.4	6.2
70–74	21.1	7.5
75–79	24.3	8.8
80–84	23.2	6.9
85+	20.0	6.3

SOURCE: Elderly Suicide Data Bases: Levels, Availability, Omission (p. 21) by J. L. McIntosh. Paper presented at the Annual Meeting of the Gerontological Society of America, San Francisco, California, November, 1983. Reprinted with permission.

among the aged should not be confused with euthanasia. It is precisely the result of confusing issues of euthanasia with those of ageism that the high potential for death by suicide among the elderly is greatly ignored.

Another component that contributes to the high risk is lack of supportive networks, which are important in predicting the outcome of bereavement. Lindeman (1949) found that survivors of the Coconut Grove fire and those who were able to deal successfully with their losses were those who had a support group. Crisis theory was based upon this research: it is important to have twenty-four-hour service where people are available and interested in helping.

In working with those who are feared to be suicidal, be honest and sincere. Do not patronize. Acknowledge your uneasiness with suicide in a calm manner. If the person has a history of suicide attempts, and/or there is a high likelihood that the suicide will take place and resources are available to carry it out, then help must be secured immediately.

Always take suicide threats seriously. Don't argue with threatening statements. Don't tell the person that there is everything to live for, and don't use paradoxical statements by saying "Okay, let's see you do it." For example, remind the older person that there are other options. Reduce environmental hazards and insure that the person is not left alone. Be familiar with organizations that can provide emergency service, such as hospitalization and treatment. Don't try to placate the suicidal individual. Things may not be getting better, and tomorrow may not be seen as any more promising than today. In the unfortunate event that a suicide attempt is made, don't blame yourself. You are not so powerful that you could force another person to kill himself or ultimately stop the person from making the attempt.

As previously stated, alcohol consumption has been correlated with suicide attempts. As many as 75 percent of suicides were attempted while under its influence. This is not surprising, since the prevalence of alcohol use among bereaved older persons is higher than among the nonbereaved elderly.

HOW CAN WE HELP THE HEALING PROCESS?

Facilitative conditions are necessary components in the helping relationship (Rogers 1962, Butler and Hansen 1973). These core conditions comprise the quality of the interpersonal encounters that are ultimately most important: they help in facilitating change, grieving, and resolution within the older person. These core conditions, which describe an attitude initially expressed by the counselor, include congruence, empathy, and unconditional positive regard.

According to Rogers (1957, 1962) genuineness is important in contributing to the formation of a therapeutic alliance. This requires the counselor to be "present," interested, and not presenting a facade deemed to be a professional demeanor.

Congruence is an important dynamic because it is portrayed to the client by several modes. Nonverbal behavior significantly demonstrates incongruence: if the older, grieving person perceives a disharmony between verbal and nonverbal messages, the counselor will not be perceived as honest, and a trusting relationship will not be established. Trust is complex and delicate. A counselor works hard to achieve it, but it *can* be destroyed by one instance of incongruence. Sincerity and honesty are important aspects in the helping relationship.

Empathy is perhaps the most widely accepted and well-known behavior in the helper's repertoire (Haase and Tepper 1972). To sense the older person's inner world "as if" it were your own is empathic or understanding. This ability to "walk in another person's shoes" is essential to a growth-producing relationship. The counselor needs to focus on the client's feelings and perceptions and zoom in to comprehend the intention without being bound up in it. Through this sensitive understanding, it is possible for the client to gain more self-understanding and awareness of the grieving process. This facilitates learning and change.

Counselors need to be aware that empathy does not involve an evaluative component. It does, however, involve a risk for the counselor since, by being open to another person's perspective, the possibility exists that the counselor's perspective may change. In dealing with the aged, the empathic condition is the most significant element in changing counselors' attitudes toward the aged.

Empathy is demonstrated through verbal and nonverbal cues (Carkhuff 1967). Older persons judge empathic messages by cues such as lean, distance, eye contact, and facial expressions (Haase and Tepper 1972). The counselor's understanding of the older person will resonate verbally and nonverbally what the client is experiencing.

Unconditional positive regard is demonstrated by a warm, positive, and accepting attitude toward the "essence" of older grieving clients and their significant others. In demonstrating this nonjudgmental attitude, the client is neither liked nor accepted on the basis of preconceived behavior that the grieving person "should" demonstrate. The total person is embraced as "special." Accepting the elderly and perceiving their capacity for growth implies respect (Dustin and George 1977).

Both verbal and nonverbal responses indicate the degree of acceptance the health care worker experiences with the elderly. Physical distancing of the person from the helper is an indicator of acceptance or nonacceptance: when an elder believes an encounter to be unacceptable, more distance will be sought.

These core conditions are pervasive in their influence toward establishing and maintaining a helping relationship. This requires that counselors engage in ongoing assessments to evaluate the intentions, responses, and nonverbal behavior of the elderly.

In determining the facilitative process, the expectations of the helpers are influenced as well. Much research has been conducted that emphasizes how expectations affect behavior. The aged, because of their innate push to self-actualize in the life review process, are easily manipulated by others' thought projections of what their decorum should be. They are generally very open to what others believe they know about them in addition to what they know about themselves. This accounts for the lack of behavior change among the elderly, despite indications that they *are* capable of making great changes (Weiner, Brok & Snodowsky 1978).

As work proceeds on this "life review," the elderly prepare for their inevitable death. Finishing one's business often requires a "bent ear," i.e., someone to listen. All too frequently, the family builds a wall of silence out of fear. References to death are ignored, considered morbid, or attributed to "senility." For the aging parent, the opportunity to ventilate anger, frustration, fear, etc., openly while preparing for death is seldom available. Grief becomes increasingly purposeful as we age, in order to evaluate our accomplishments, grieve our losses, and prepare for our final loss—death.

The following poem, written by an eighty-year-old woman on a psychogeriatric floor demonstrates this life review process. Imagine what wonderful things could have happened, had her writings been found while she was alive!

> What do you see Nurses,
>   What do you see?
> Are you thinking
>   When you are looking at me
> A crabby old woman,
>   Not very wise,
> Uncertain of habit—
>   With far away eyes,
> Who dribbles her food
>   And makes no reply,
> When you say in a loud voice
>   "I do wish you'd try."
> Who seems not to notice
>   The things that you do,
> And forever is losing
>   A stocking or shoe.
> Who unresisting or not,
>   Lets you do as you will
> With bathing and feeding,
>   The long day to fill.
> Is that what you're thinking,
>   Is that what you see?
> Then open your eyes Nurse,
>   You are not looking at me.
> I'll tell you who I am
>   As I sit here so still;
> As I use at your bidding,

As I eat at your will,
I'm a small child of ten
    With a Father and Mother,
Brothers and Sisters who
    Love one another.
A young girl of sixteen,
    With wings on her feet
Dreaming that soon now
    A lover she'll meet:
A Bride soon at twenty,
    My heart gives a leap,
Remembering the vows
    That I promised to keep:
At twenty-five now
    I have young of my own
Who need me to build
    A secure happy home.
A woman of thirty,
    My young now grow fast,
Bound to each other
    With ties that should last;
At forty my young sons
    Now grown and will all be gone
But my man stays beside me
    To see I don't mourn.
At fifty once more
    Babies play around my knee,
Again we know children,
    My loved one and me.
Dark days are upon me,
    My husband is dead,
I look at the future
    I shudder with dread,
For my young are all busy
    Rearing young of their own,
And I think of the years
    And the love that I've known.
I'm an old woman now
    And nature is cruel,
Tis her jest to make
    Old age look like a fool.
The body it crumbles,

Grace and vigor depart,
There is now a stone
Where once I had a heart:
But inside this old carcass
A young girl still dwells
And now and again
My battered heart swells.
I remember the joys,
I remember the pain,
And I'm loving and living
Life over again.
I think of the years
All too few gone too fast,
And accept the stark fact
That nothing can last.
So open your eyes nurses,
Open and see,
Not a crabby old woman,
Look closer, see ME.

The helper's attitude and expectations have tremendous influence over the relationship with the mature grieving person. It is very important that this power be acknowledged and dealt with responsibly. It is a travesty that society does not embrace this fact: direct care providers (e.g., nurses aides and maintenance personnel) are not addressed for their very important impact on the "being" of the elder.

When the counselor feels comfortable in dealing with the losses that the elderly experience, support techniques can help facilitate the grieving process. These techniques include encouraging the expression of feelings, honest reassurance, emphasizing the positive, recognizing progress, and, when appropriate, directing interests outside of the self.

It is always important for the counselor to recognize that not all people react in the same way. Don't push: let the older person and/or the family set the pace. Most grieving persons need reassurance that their "style" is normal. Grieving is painful and it takes time. People need to be reassured they are not going "crazy," since this is the reason many give for seeking counseling for bereavement.

Permission to grieve and to recognize losses is important. Grief has a cumulative nature. If griefwork is not done, the feelings remain dormant. When another loss is experienced that grief may combine with previous feelings. As more losses are shelved, the grief grows larger and larger, causing grief "overload," a term coined by Robert Kastenbaum. Help involves recognizing the losses and grieving them. Being supportive and caring facilitates a healthy reintegration.

Management of grief in the aged is important. The same fears and taboos that prohibit the discussion of life events and preparations for death also inhibit the help for those who mourn. People don't know what to say, or believe they will "unnecessarily" remind the bereaved of the loss. Of course, the notion of the person forgetting is minimal. It is not what is said that is helpful, but the mere fact that others are there with the older bereaved person. This is what consoles. It is focusing on and expressing the pain of grief that eventually abates and gives new dimension. In recognizing, coping with, and integrating the grief experience, growth will occur.

Paramount in assisting the healthful grief process is the manner in which subsequent losses are brought to the attention of the older person and significant others. Announcing a loss is a difficult task for those in the helping professions. It is also a difficult experience to learn of yet another loss. There are methods that help to make this more natural, methods that may facilitate the grieving process.

When giving the information, sit down and achieve eye-to-eye contact with the person(s). If you are responsible for the helping relationship, go yourself. Don't send someone whom he/she doesn't know. Whenever possible, have someone go who is significant to the person, someone who can stay and offer support. Make the environment as conducive as possible to giving the person permission to express feelings. Encouraging the venting of emotion is an important dynamic in supportive work. Emphasize the positive wherever possible. Be cautious, however, not to minimize the significance of the event. Soften the initial blow by using words that do not dramatize the event or traumatize the bereaved.

HELPING THE DYING PROCESS

A study conducted by Youngs-Brockupp identified information and hope as the two most important areas of help to persons who are dying. However, giving people (and especially the older person) information about their health and exploring hope is, sadly to say, very seldom done.

In the name of love and caring, important information is often withheld regarding a person's physical condition and its implications. The giving of information is vital in developing and maintaining an open atmosphere. Repeatedly, older people identify having information about themselves as a right! Research indicates that only relatively few elderly people (approximately 3 percent) do not wish to be informed of a life-threatening condition. In most instances, people *do want to know*. Adult children, as well as health care providers and workers, rarely realize the strength of parents who experience failing health. The older persons, with the family present, should be given the information, which will help to establish open lines of communication.

Families also need to have information and support during the dying process. They need to know that the dying elderly persons do have control over their arena. The dying person may want to be with loved family members and friends at the time of death. Then again, the individual may want to be alone, thus sparing the significant others; or the person may not want to be touched during the process. For some, it is important that they be given permission to let go. These issues are difficult for family members to understand. Guidance and support is needed through this important transition. To let go of a person you love and who has loved you is never easy at any age.

Fanslow (1988) identifies a process in the hope system. She points out how rarely we are asked what our hopes are or how extremely rare it is to ask older persons about their hopes. This is sad, considering it is the second most important aspect in dealing with a loss. The hope system, as Fanslow postulates it, includes the following:

1. The hope that everything will be better, that there will be a cure, or that things will return to normal.

2. There will be hope for a treatment that will be effective. Maybe something will happen to help the situation to return to normal; things will be the same or better.

3. The hope that life will be prolonged to allow for more quality time.

4. The hope that death will be peaceful and on the dying person's terms. There will be an absence of pain, both physically and mentally.

Most older persons do not fear death; rather, they fear the process of dying—the pain and loneliness. With our current technical knowledge, we can be assured that no one need die in pain. Advances in palliation (pain control) can insure living with awareness and without pain. Unfortunately, due to the values of many in the health profession, palliation is a threat.

This means not giving comfort measures because the caregivers do not want to recognize that the older person is dying. Many professionals in the medical field view death as a failure. They are in the field to make people better. Palliative measures connote giving up, not treating aggressively. Symptom management will not cure or treat the individual; therefore, it is not valued, and persons continue to die in pain unnecessarily.

Older people die primarily in hospitals, although most people hope to die in their homes or among persons they know and care for. In many long-term care facilities, the dying are transferred to a hospital, due to the regulatory agency mandates. There the elderly die, among unfamiliar staff who may or may not have had time to attend to their needs.

It is also important to consider the spiritual needs of the aged who are dying. Belief and hope in what death means and what lies in store for us after death serves to shape our understanding of death. Nancy Little Fox in *The Joy of Geriatrics* writes of how important it is to hold the person's hand and join in prayer. In our technical society, such needs are often overlooked. The religious, spiritual, cultural, and ethnic dimensions of the whole person are negated, leading to fragmented care. In addressing these spiritual needs, it is important to respect the cultural and ethnic values of the older person, the family members, and your own needs.

The most important transition from life to death can be helped by creating a supportive and loving environment. The use of familiar and restful music, meaningful discussions, and a peaceful atmosphere can facilitate the ultimate letting go. In Fanslow's *Healing the Dying,* family members and counselors are given exercises that produce relaxation in the dying person. These exercises utilize therapeutic touch. Family members and counselors can become actively involved in the process of making it the ultimate act of loving and caring. It is indeed a beautiful ending to the final chapter.

WHAT CAN WE LEARN ABOUT LIVING FROM THE AGED WHO ARE DYING?

In the song "The Rose," the notion is put forth ". . . it's the soul afraid of dying that never learns to live." Workers in the field of death and dying say this is true. When we face physical mortality, it forces us to review our lives. In assessing what is important to us, stating our real priorities, we cut out many of the unnecessary tasks. We look more at the aspects of our lives that really matter.

Persons who are near death, those who have had after-death experiences, and those who have survived the loss of a loved one, strongly believe in the dynamic of "keeping current." This means telling the persons that you love that you love them. It means telling them how proud and happy you are as a result of a kind gesture or an accomplishment. Not living in the moment makes grieving difficult. A bereaved girl who was a patient of Dr. Elizabeth Kübler-Ross wrote a letter to her dead boyfriend as part of her therapy to keep current. It reads:

A woman wrote to Vietnam:
Remember the day I borrowed your brand new car and I dented it?
I thought you would kill me but you didn't.
Remember the time I dragged you to the beach and you said it would
   rain and it did?
I thought you would say I told you so. But you didn't.
And the time I flirted with all the guys to make you jealous and you
   were.
I thought you would leave me, but you didn't.
And the time I spilled blueberry pie all over your brand new car rug.
   I thought you would drop me for sure, but you didn't.
And the time I forgot to tell you the dance was formal and you showed
   up in blue jeans. I thought you would smack me, but you didn't.
And there were so many things I wanted to make up to you when
   you returned from Vietnam, but you didn't.

Those who live life on the principle of being current, speak of the richness and fullness of life. The knowledge that one is prepared for death takes much guilt out of the way in enjoying and experiencing the path of one's life. Living in the "here and now" also gives life a special meaning. After all, the only time we have to react is at the present. You can't live in the past.

The aged who are dying may offer perspectives on life's priorities. Accomplishments are seen as minor points in a lifetime. Many say that families, loving, and caring are seen as the great gifts in their lives.

In listening to the review of the elders, we gain perspective for today. Only in this way can we avoid the pitfalls of yesteryear. By gaining from the wisdom of the dying, we can realize the important tasks of living, loving, and making our own transition when the time comes.

FOR DISCUSSION

1. What are the different types of losses and what factors affect the depth, length, and intensity of the grieving process?
2. What factors facilitate the healing process?
3. What role do hope and information play in the grief/healing process?
4. How are dreams involved in the grieving process?
5. What do the dying teach the living about life?
6. What aspects are involved in a lethality assessment if suicide is suspected?

BIBLIOGRAPHY

Assimacopoulos, L. "Realizing Empathy in Loss." *Journal of Psychosocial Nursing in Mental Health Service* 25, no. 11 (November 1987): 26-29.

Baker, H. M. "Some Thoughts on Helping Grieving Families." *Journal of Emergency Nursing* 13, no. 6 (November/December 1987): 359-362.

Carkhuff, R. "Toward a Comprehensive Model of Facilitative Interpersonal Processes." *Journal of Counseling Psychology* 14 (1967): 67-72.

Cohen, G. D. "Mental Health Services and the Elderly: Needs and Options." *American Journal of Psychology* 133 (1976): 65-68.

Dunlop, Richard S. *Helping the Bereaved.* Philadelphia: The Charles Press Publishers, Inc., 1978.

Dustin, R., and George, R. *Action Counseling for Behavior Change* (2d. ed.). Rhode Island: Carroll Press, 1977.

Fanslow, C. *Healing the Dying.* Presentation at Pumpkin Hollow, 1988.

———. "Therapeutic Touch: A Healing Modality Through Life." *Topics in Clinical Nursing* (July 1983).

———. "Therapeutic Touch and the Elderly." Paper presented at Pediatric Roundtable #10 on Touch, 1983.

Freeman, L. *The Sorrow and the Fury.* Englewood Cliffs, N.J.: Prentice-Hall, Inc., 1988.

Haase, R., and Tepper, D. "Nonverbal Components of Pathic Communication." *Journal of Counseling Psychology* 19 (1972): 417-424.

Kübler-Ross, E. *On Death and Dying.* New York: Macmillan Publishing Co., 1974.

Lindeman, E. "Symptomatology and Management of Acute Grief." *American Journal of Psychiatry* 101 (1949): 141.

Osgood, N. J. *Suicide in the Elderly.* Rockville, Md.: Aspen Publishers, 1985.

Pincus, L. *Death and the Family.* New York: Pantheon Books, 1974.

Raphael, B. *The Anatomy of Bereavement.* New York: Basic Books, 1983.

Rogers, C. "The Necessary and Sufficient Conditions of Therapeutic Personality Change." *Journal of Counseling Psychology* (1957): 95-103.

———. "The Interpersonal Relationship." *Harvard Educational Review* (Fall 1962): 416-429.

Siegel, B. S. *Love, Medicine, and Miracles.* New York: Harper & Row Publishers, 1986.

Silverstone, B., and Hyman H. K. *You and Your Aging.* New York: Panther Books, 1982.

Sullender, R. .S *Grief and Growth.* New York: The Paulist Press, 1985.

Warden, J. W. *Grief Counseling and Grief Therapy: A Handbook for the Mental Health Practitioner.* New York: Springer Publishing Co., 1982.

Weiner, M. .B., Brok, A., and Snodowsky, A. *Working with the Aged.* Englewood Cliffs, N.J.: Prentice-Hall, 1978.

Contributors

RICHELLE N. CUNNINGHIS, Ed.M., OTR, is the executive director of Geriatric Educational Consultants in Willingboro, New Jersey, and an adjunct assistant professor in the School of Allied Health Sciences at Temple University. She has authored works on documentation, reality activities, and a guide and a programming handbook for activities coordinators. Ms. Cunninghis has given workshops on these and related topics to professionals throughout the United States.

ELIZABETH S. DEICHMAN, Ed.M., OTR, FAOTA, is president of Potentials Development for Health and Aging Services in Buffalo, New York, a firm specializing in publications for activity professionals. As research clinical assistant professor at the State University of New York at Buffalo, she pioneered the development of courses on communicating with and serving elderly adults. Ms. Deichman has published and lectured extensively on these topics throughout the United States, Canada, and England. For the past two decades her publications and conference/workshop topics have focused on the importance of meaningful and rewarding activities as one grows older.

MARIAN DEUTSCHMAN, Ph.D., is assistant professor of public communication at the State University of New York College at Buffalo. She has more than fifteen years' experience as an organizational design consultant for institutional and corporate settings, and her extensive background as a trainer in the areas of the physical environment and communication behavior is utilized in workshops and conferences throughout the United States and Canada.

DAVID DUBE, M.D., is medical director of St. Camillus Health and Rehabilitation Facility, in addition to which he serves on the clinical faculty in the Division of Geriatrics at the State University of New York Health Sciences Center in Syracuse. He has co-authored articles on many topics pertinent to geriatrics: tuberculosis, nutrition, and assessment in consultation format.

DELLVINA GROSS, Ph.D., OTR, FAOTA, is associate professor and director of graduate programs in the Department of Occupational Therapy at Temple University. She has extensive experience consulting and working with the elderly.

DORIS B. HAMMOND, Ph.D., is a guidance counselor for Aiken County School District and adjunct professor of psychology at the University of South Carolina. She is a certified professional counselor and sex counselor.

MARY V. KIRCHHOFER, B.S., OTR, is retired vice-president of Potentials Development for Health and Aging Services. She has been instrumental in obtaining grant funding for an Independent Living Project in the Buffalo area, and has organized and directed a Seniors Center and an Adult Day Care Center.

REGINA KOCIECKI, B.A., is assistant to the chair (emeritus) of the Department of Occupational Therapy at the State University of New York at Buffalo. She also serves as an editorial associate with Potentials Development for Health and Aging Services. As a retiree she remains politically active in areas of interest to retired persons.

ROSEMARY MCCASLIN, Ph.D., ACSW, is assistant professor in the School of Social Welfare at the University of California at Berkeley. For the past fourteen years, her research and publications have focused on social services for the elderly.

MARJORIE PLUMB, Ph.D., is associate professor emeritus of the School of Medicine at the State University of New York at Buffalo. She is currently in private practice as a clinical psychologist.

KENT NELSON TIGGES, M.S., OTR., FAOTA, is associate professor of occupational therapy at the State University of New York at Buffalo and director of occupational therapy for Hospice Buffalo, Inc. He has lectured extensively in England, Scotland, South Africa, and Canada on theory of practice, professional roles and responsibilities, and terminal cancer.

DEBORAH WILKINSON-TJOA, M.S., R.N., CRC, is on the faculty of the Interdisciplinary Social Services Department at the State University of New York at Buffalo, where she instructs in social gerontology, death and dying, and community mental health. In addition, she is a consultant with the Life and Death Transition Center, Inc., the Center for the Study of Aging, and Potentials Development in Health and Aging Services.

CONNIE ZUCKERMAN, J.D., is an assistant professor in the Department of Epidemiology and Social Medicine at the Albert Einstein College of Medicine at the Bronx Municipal Center. She is also a consultant on legal and ethical issues at the Montefiore Medical Center in New York and at the Long Island Jewish Medical Center. Ms. Zuckerman has been involved in numerous studies examining the medical decision-making process of elderly individuals and has lectured and published extensively on the rights of elderly persons in the health care area.

DATE DUE

JUN 1 1 2003	

DATE DUE

NOV 0 9 2004	